YOUR VITAMINS ARE OBSOLETE

The Vitamer Revolution: A Program for Healthy Living and Healthy Longevity

Sheldon Zablow, M.D.

HybridGlobal
PUBLISHING

Published by
Hybrid Global Publishing
301 East 57th Street
4th Floor
New York, NY 10022

Manufactured in the United States of America, or in the United Kingdom when distributed elsewhere.

Zablow, Sheldon
> Your Vitamins are Obsolete: The Vitamer Revolution: A Program for Healthy Living and Healthy Longevity
> LCCN: 2019915145
> ISBN: 978-1-948181-86-0
> eBook: 978-1-948181-87-7

Cover design by: Jonathan Pleska
Copyediting and interior design by: Claudia Volkman
Author photo by: Connie Villa
Illustrations by: Steve Cook

Disclaimer: This book publication and associated website contains the opinions and ideas of its author. It is intended to present useful and educational material on the subjects addressed. The book is sold with the understanding that the author and the publisher are not engaged in rendering medical, health, or any other kind of personal professional services in this book. The reader should consult a medical professional before embracing any of the suggestions in this book or drawing any inferences from it. The author and the publisher specifically disclaim all responsibility for any liability, loss or risk personal or otherwise that might be incurred as a consequence, directly or indirectly, of the use and application of any of the contents in this book and website. SZMD

www.sheldonzablowmd.com

DEDICATION

To Jane E. Brody, who reduces suffering with her words.

CONTENTS

PREFACE

Genetics, Surgery, Stress, Hormones, GERD Medications, Metformin, Aging, Pollution, Weight Gain, Voluntary and Involuntary Veganism, Poorly Manufactured Supplements →↓B_{12}/Folate

↓B_{12}/Folate →↓Epigenetic Methylation →↓Gene Suppression (↑Expression of Pro-Inflammatory Genes) →↑Chronic Inflammation →↓Healthy Living (Dementia, Diabetes, Heart Disease, Cancer)

Your Vitamins Are Obsolete tells the story of why certain vitamins found in our supplements or purchased individually do not fulfill all the expectations we have of them. To explain this obsolescence, this book will focus on the two most essential vitamins that facilitate the creation of the fuel molecules used by cells for energy, cleanse the cells of waste products, and modulate the expression of genes—B_{12} and folate.

There are many steps and obstacles along the way for vitamins found in the soil and in plants to get all the way to your cells through diet. When multivitamins are used, there are additional challenges for the body to metabolize the synthetic B vitamins found in most supplements into the bioactive vitamer forms required.

In the title, *Vitamins* is shorthand for "multiple vitamin supplements" that are obsolete. Multivitamins are taken to achieve a health benefit or as inexpensive health insurance—insurance against a possible missing nutrient in the diet that could contribute to any one of a number of signs and symptoms.

There are thousands of nutrient combinations available, but not all of the ingredients in these multivitamin arrangements play together well. Current supplements can provide benefits for many people, with some individual nutrients being better absorbed than others. People should continue to take their multivitamins for whatever current benefits they might provide, keeping in mind that after finishing this book, you will be well aware of the pitfalls and the better choices available.

The book will focus on the two most essential vitamins—B_{12} and folate—in their vitamer forms. A vitamer is one of many molecular forms of a particular vitamin. I will be using the term to specifically focus on the bioactive forms (vitamers), which are the only ones that cells can use. I call these B vitamers the most essential of the essential nutrients because if there is not enough B_{12} and folate, the use of other vitamins and other medical interventions are not biologically efficient. For example, you could have plenty of vitamin D and calcium, but if you don't have enough of these B_{12} and folate vitamers, you can still develop osteoporosis.

Energy is required by every cell to complete all the other thousands of biochemical reactions in the most efficient manner possible. Low intake or utilization of B_{12} and folate causes reduced cellular energy, which slows cognitive function, increases fatigue, worsens sleep, and causes mood disturbances. Worst of all, a deficiency of either increases chronic inflammation which contributes to the onset of most major illnesses. The connection between sub-adequate vitamer levels and chronic inflammation through the field of epigenetics is *The Vitamer Revolution*—the science behind the future of medicine.

As the chapters unfold, the new knowledge you will acquire can help you make better choices for yourself and your loved ones and save your dollars from being merely flushed away. By the end of the book, you will fully understand the importance of vitamers and how to use them for healthy living and healthy longevity.

The COVID-19 pandemic was expanding as this book was finalized. For updates on the connection between viral illness progression, homocysteine, and vitamers, please visit:

sheldonzablowmd.com

INTRODUCTION

VITAMIN OR VITAMER?

↓Vitamers →↓Epigenetic Methylation →
↑Inflammatory Load→↑Unhealthy Aging

The vitamins you take are obsolete, as is the entire $25 billion supplement industry. This obsolescence doesn't only cost you money, it can markedly ramp up your risk of suffering from serious illness. How does it do this and what else do you need to know to truly promote your health?

As a psychiatric physician, treating patients with a wide variety of mental health problems, I often note a physical health overlay; that is, my patients typically suffer from medical conditions in addition to their psychological ones. Trying to fully understand the connection between the two in one of my patients took me on a path of new insights.

In 2006, I started my search for an answer—any answer—to my growing concern about a female patient whose physical health had deteriorated despite the best efforts of her medical team. What I learned surprised me, and when I applied these new lessons to other patients, they benefited in ways none of us predicted.

When I first consulted with Susan, she was a forty-year-old professional needing treatment for anxiety and depression triggered by work-related stress. From a treatment perspective, Susan's case appeared pretty straightforward. Although overweight, she looked healthy. After doing some hard work in psychotherapy, including the intermittent use of medication, Susan emerged from her emotional difficulties, and her usual good mood returned. Not long afterward, she was diagnosed as prediabetic and decided to reduce her risk of developing full-blown diabetes by undergoing gastric bypass surgery.

The surgery was a success. Susan's weight dropped, and her cholesterol, blood sugar, and other measures of health improved considerably. She felt physically well, increased her exercise, and was in good spirits for several months. Then slowly her energy level and mood began declining. Oddly enough, she also seemed to be aging at an accelerated rate, looking older than her years. This was puzzling because apart from the successful surgery and weight loss, everything else in her life was the same. I asked about her marriage, work, medications, laboratory tests, exercise regimen, relationships with family and friends, and more—anything that might explain her physical and emotional decline—but nothing stood out. Her other physicians and I simply could not understand why her health was declining so rapidly.

On a hunch, I asked her to bring in all of her medications and supplements so I could look them over. Until that moment, I had never read the labels on any patient's vitamin bottles—or on my own, for that matter—so I wasn't sure what I was looking for. I was immediately struck by the fact Susan's multivitamin tablets contained 8,333 percent of the RDA (Recommended Dietary Allowance) for vitamin B12. Why so much? Shouldn't 100 percent be enough? I also noticed the vitamin B12 in her supplement was in the cyanocobalamin form, and I remembered from medical school that this is an artificial form of B12.

As I began to study up on vitamins and nutrition, I realized how little we were taught about these subjects in medical school. I did remember learning the body has a three-year backup supply of B12 in the liver (which I later discovered is false) and that, with our modern abundance of food and supplements, there is little concern about running short of this vitamin (also false). I understood at that time B12's classic deficiency disease, megaloblastic anemia, was very rare, easy to spot, and just as easy to treat. If a deficiency is identified, we were told, a standard multivitamin pill or B12 injection as a "quick boost" is typically all that is necessary. In short, we were given to understand the lack of B12 and other vitamins just wasn't an issue in the modern world.

As I continued studying up on vitamins, I wondered why folate, another of the B vitamins, was commonly formulated as folic acid in supplements. Like cyanocobalamin, folic acid is a man-made form of the vitamin, not the naturally occurring form found in food and utilized by the human body. I had no idea whether these artificial forms were as good as the "real thing" or might be harmful, at least to some people. I wanted to find out. And the more I researched the matter, the more interesting it became.

What Are Vitamins, Exactly?

Once scientists determined there were special substances in food, they called them vitamins and sought to define them. Although they understood vitamins were essential to human survival, their exact functions remained unclear. For example, vitamins aren't used to build bodily structures in the same way the mineral calcium is used to build bones, yet bones and other structures cannot be built without vitamins. So what are they, exactly? The reference textbook titled *The Vitamins: Fundamental Aspects in Nutrition and Health*, Fourth Edition, edited by Dr. Gerald F. Combs, provides an excellent history and definition of vitamins. It says that a vitamin:

- is an organic compound distinct from fats, carbohydrates, and proteins
- is a natural component of foods in which it is present in small amounts
- is essential, also in minute amounts, for normal physiologic function (i.e., maintenance, growth, development, reproduction)
- causes, by its absence or underutilization, a specific deficiency syndrome
- is not synthesized in the host in amounts adequate to meet normal physiologic needs

Putting it all together, then, a vitamin is an organic compound, a micronutrient naturally present in foods and essential in very small amounts for normal bodily functions and disease prevention. It is also a substance the body cannot make on its own—or, at least, the body can't manufacture this substance in sufficient amounts to maintain health. (We photosynthesize vitamin D.) The required mineral micronutrients in our diet are inorganic elements like calcium, magnesium, iron, etc.

Vital Vitamers

One of the most important things I learned during the course of my studies is that vitamins come in many forms, and those found in supplements are not necessarily the kinds the body uses for basic cellular functions. Instead, modern vitamins are constructed from man-made artificial compounds. These artificial varieties must be processed by the body and converted into biologically active structures that can be referred to as *vitamers* (pronounced VY-TA-MURS). Only then can they be utilized to optimize the function of each and every cell in the body. Unfortunately for the consumer, the vitamers of B_{12} and folate (the bioactive forms) are not found in most supplements; only the synthetic molecules are used.[1]

The B_{12} molecule exists in essentially four different configurations, each differentiated by the attachment of an additional, smaller molecule. The two naturally occurring, bioactive vitamers in animals are called *adenosylcobalamin* (A-B_{12}) because of its adenosyl attachment, and *methylcobalamin* (M-B_{12}) because of its methyl attachment. You can think of these as the "vitamer forms."

Manufacturers transformed the naturally occurring vitamers into cheaper man-made vitamins by adding one harmless cyanide molecule. The result is the artificial *cyanocobalamin* (C-B_{12}), the chemical found in almost all of our supplements. Now the body must convert C-B_{12} back into one of the vitamer forms before it can be used. The fourth form, *hydroxocobalamin* (H-B_{12}), so named because of its hydroxyl attachment, is manufactured by bacteria "in the wild" or by bacteria in a factory, and it is the form often used for injections. It, too, must be converted by the body into one of the bioactive forms before the body can use it.

Sample Supplemental Facts on Bottle Similar to Susan's

Supplement Facts

Serving Size: 1 Tablet Servings Per Container: 30

	Amount Per Tablet	% Daily Value
Vitamin B6 (as pyridoxine HCl)	5mg	250%
Folate (as folic acid)	400 mcg	100%
Vitamin B12 (cyanocobalamin)	1000 mcg	16,667%
Biotin	25 mcg	8%

---

[1] B_{12} and folate are not the only vitamers of vitamins, and there is some variation in definitions. The word can be used to signify all forms of a vitamin, but it is also used to signify the naturally occurring bioactive forms. For the purposes of this book, vitamer refers to the bioactive forms.

Right in the middle of my literature research, I stumbled upon the probable reason Susan was ingesting 8,333 percent (others take 16,667 percent) of the RDA for B12 and was still not getting enough: Only about 1 percent at most of the C-B12 form found in her supplements can be absorbed by the body. That's because the artificial C-B12 absorption relies on an inefficient process called passive diffusion. If you do the math, you'll see the massive amount of C-B12 in the supplement actually provided her body with at most only 83 percent of the RDA (1 percent of 8,333 percent). So, even if Susan's passive diffusion process was working perfectly, the vitamins were made perfectly, and her body was absorbing the maximum amount possible, she would still fall 17 percent behind the RDA every day. Relying solely on these kinds of supplements for her B12 intake, Susan would have to take more than 10,000 percent of the RDA just to stay even. And if she didn't, within a short period of time, she could be very much behind and showing early subclinical (that is, not detectable by the usual tests) signs of B12 deficiency.

I then realized by trying to get her B12 by taking a multivitamin, Susan was making her problem worse. Multivitamin manufacturers typically combine vitamin C and iron with the B12, all in one tablet. Unfortunately, these substances tend to bind together to form a macromolecule—a very large molecule—the body cannot absorb.[2] When they are not absorbed, the vitamins are eventually flushed away. Susan might not absorb any B12 at all despite the manufacturer's claim of 8,333 percent RDA.

What You and Your Doctor Don't Know Can Hurt You

Although I could have devoted this book to the function and importance of every vitamin, I decided to focus on B12 and folate for two reasons. First, both vitamins are vital for maintaining cellular energy and cellular hygiene and both influence the way DNA is expressed. Second, a deficiency of either vitamin can cause significant problems body-wide, including permanent nerve damage, memory problems, fatigue, and depression. And yet these two nutrients are generally overlooked as the causes of these maladies. Symptoms typically have to be severe before a doctor will test for a B12 or folate deficiency. Even when a deficiency is diagnosed, the prescribed treatments are likely to fail. Why? It all boils down to one major issue: Few healthcare professionals and patients understand the difference between vitamins and vitamers. This lack of knowledge about B12 and folate puts millions at grave risk for serious

---

[2]Gerald F. Combs, *The Vitamins: Fundamental Aspects in Nutrition and Health, Fourth Edition* (Amsterdam: Elsevier Academic Press, 2012), p. 379.

problems. Below are some little-known facts I will explore in the chapters to follow:

- Most medical training and textbooks state that there is a three-year reserve of B12 in the liver. All healthcare is based on this incorrect assumption. The liver does not and cannot store *water-soluble* B vitamins. Many medical treatments could be more effective if this B12 challenge was addressed and proactive B12 initiated.

- Only 30 to 40 percent of people have enough of the enzyme that efficiently converts the folic acid found in supplements and grain products into folate, the bioactive form used by the body.

- Bioavailability of folate from a wide variety of foods varies widely. (The percentage of a substance ingested that actually works is its bioavailability.) Spinach has a high iron content but a low iron bioavailability because we can't digest it out of the plant fiber.

- There is plenty of B12 and folate in red meat, but 50 percent of people over the age of fifty cannot manufacture enough stomach acid to break down the protein to release these vitamers.

- The widespread use of medications to reduce stomach acids, such as H-2 blockers and proton-pump inhibitors, can lead to a medically induced B12 deficiency, as can the exposure to nitrous oxide anesthesia used for surgical and dental procedures.

- The enzyme that changes folic acid into bioactive folate, known as MTHFR, is blocked by many medications, including NSAIDs, antibiotics, diuretics, aspirin, birth control pills, hormone replacement therapy, steroids, and metformin.

- The damage to sensory nerve cells due to B12 deficiency starts long before the shortage can be detected on blood tests for the vitamer-deficient anemia called macrocytic anemia.

- Deficiencies in B12 or folate are not nearly as rare or as easy to diagnose as we were led to believe in medical training.

Perhaps the best way to explain the amazing potential of vitamers is with this picture of the famous "agouti gene mice"—famous to laboratory researchers, that is.

The smaller mouse on the right is very healthy, with brown hair and a slim, muscular body. He was delivered by a mother who had been fed a proper mouse

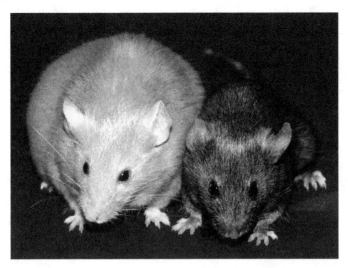

(Image by R. Jirtle/ D. Dolinoy 2007 and used in compliance with Creative Commons attribution 3.0 unported license)

diet, complete with all the necessary vitamers. In contrast, the genetically identical mouse on the left is terribly obese, at great risk of developing dementia, diabetes, and heart disease, and sporting a very unnatural-looking yellowish coat. He was born to a mother having been deliberately deprived of folate. The absence of this one vitamer was all it took to set up entire litters for lifetimes of disease by changing the way their genes behaved. How this happens is a subject we'll talk more about in future chapters. I want you to see this now, so you will understand good health is not just a matter of popping a multivitamin pill you've picked up in the grocery store. The vitamers you do or do not ingest every day are positioning you—and your descendants—for good health or disease.

Are We Overlooking Deficiency Symptoms?

As I sat and tried to absorb all of this information, I wondered if a lack of B_{12} or folate might be responsible for Susan's problems. I knew gastric bypass procedures such as the one Susan underwent interfered with her body's ability to absorb these two nutrients, as well as others. It's quite likely her other doctors had not considered this possibility, for their understanding of vitamin B deficiencies were probably as limited as mine. They looked no further than the standard signs and symptoms of vitamin B_{12} and folate deficiencies, as delineated by the National Institutes of Health:

Vitamin B12 Deficiency	Folate Deficiency
Anemia	Anemia
Fatigue	Fatigue
Diarrhea	Gray Hair
Bleeding gums	Mouth sores
Red, swollen tongue	Irritability
Pale skin	
Problems concentrating	
Shortness of breath (mostly with exercise)	
Constipation	
Light-headedness when standing up	
Confusion	
Dementia	
Depression	
Loss of balance	
Numbness; tingling of hands and feet	

It's interesting to note that these signs and symptoms are all easy to detect. Anemia can be identified with a simple blood test. If you happen to be suffering from one or more of the others, you'll know it—and so will your friends and family members. By the time these problems are observed, the deficiency will have already done serious damage to your health at the cellular and genetic levels. For example, if a B12 deficiency is causing numbness and tingling in your hands or feet, you may have already suffered permanent nerve damage.

This raises an obvious question: How many people are currently suffering from overlooked deficiencies of B12 or folate? Millions? Tens of millions? No one knows for sure, because no one is truly looking. Instead of waiting until trouble strikes—trouble that is perhaps irreversible—we should be looking for indications of a deficiency, which can range from tiny inefficiencies at the subcellular level all the way to obvious clinical symptoms. Here's how a combined B12/folate deficiency list might look if we included the "too small to be obvious" problems as well as the "large" problems. Do you or yours experience any of these?

- Neurologic problems—numbness, weakness, incontinence, dementia

- Cardiovascular damage—arteriosclerosis, heart attacks, strokes, pulmonary emboli

- Immune system weakness—chronic inflammation, poor wound healing, feeling sickly
- Hematologic impairment—anemia, fatigue, increased infection, poor wound healing
- Endocrinologic upset—weight gain, obesity, diabetes, osteoporosis
- Gynecologic impairment—false abnormal pap smears, PMS, postpartum depression, infertility
- Psychiatric distress—irritability, depression, anxiety, poor concentration
- Gastrointestinal problems—weight loss or gain, constipation, irritable bowel, mouth ulcers

My patient Susan certainly suffered from some of these symptoms. Knowing that the artificial forms of B12 and folate don't work consistently or at all and the bypass reduced her absorption ability, I decided to offer her a new option. At that time, there was a new FDA-approved prescription supplement containing B vitamins, categorized as a "medicinal food." Susan agreed to take the supplement faithfully for at least a month. After some positive results, she continued for several more months and eventually became a thinner and more vibrant version of herself. She told me her hair and nails had thickened. This indicated a positive protein synthesis occurring throughout her entire body.

Susan's success encouraged me to continue studying B12 and folate, as well as their relationship to genes, inflammation, and more. Other patients trying the vitamers with additional medical conditions also responded well. I learned how these nutrients helped us evolve into modern humans and how they continue to be vital to our physical and mental health today. Unfortunately, few of us are getting enough of these vitamers, and few physicians are aware of the dangers posed by this failure. So, we as a nation continue to suffer from unnecessary diseases and conditions ranging from fatigue all the way to heart disease, cancer, dementia, and unhealthy aging.

I decided to write this book to increase awareness of the tremendous impact B12 and folate have on our health, the difficulty we have in getting adequate amounts of them, and the resulting dire consequences when we don't get enough. Mastering this information can be a bit of a challenge, so don't worry if you feel a little overwhelmed by some of the terms you'll come across; you can always come back to them later. Soldier on, keeping the main points in mind. It will be well worth your effort, if for no other reason than you'll stop flushing your money down the toilet and harming your health by taking obsolete supplements. The following are some additional little-known facts that will also be explored:

- B_{12} and folate deficiency hamper the elimination of a cellular waste product called homocysteine. A buildup of homocysteine causes increased blood viscosity, blood clots, inflammation, arterial damage, unhealthy aging, and other medical problems.

- B_{12} and folate vitamers modulate the level of long-term inflammation through a process called DNA epigenetic methylation. This process regulates the protein expression of genes.

- Many textbooks are mistaken in stating the liver has the highest concentration of B_{12} in the body. It certainly has the greatest *amount* of B_{12} because it is so large, but the pituitary gland contains a much greater *concentration* of the vitamer.[3] This little-known fact has tremendous implications for health and disease because the pituitary helps regulate most hormone production in the body.

- Japan sets a high level for normal B_{12} below which neurologic symptoms start while in the US, we set the level two to three times lower at the level below which anemia starts. This means that sensory nerve damage starts before anemia changes even appear in the lab tests your doctor ordered.

- Folate and B_{12} are co-enzymes, so both must be present in adequate amounts for a few essential biochemical reactions to work, such as cellular energy production.

- Vaccinations, such as the pneumococcal vaccines, can be significantly less effective when vitamin B levels are reduced.[4]

- The availability of B_{12} is most likely the biochemical vehicle by which population growth is ultimately controlled.

- When B vitamers are taken by vegans and vegetarians, they can actually maximize the benefits of their dietary choices and reduce fertility difficulties.

---

[3]Combs, *The Vitamins,* p. 382.
[4]Fata, FT, et al, "Impaired Antibody Responses to Pneumococcal Polysaccharide in Elderly Patients with Low Serum Vitamin B_{12} Levels," *Annals of Internal Medicine,* February 1, 1996, 124(3):299-304.

- Regular use of B vitamers decreases the craving for red meat, promoting personal health and ecologic benefits.

- Only humans have a high concentration of methyl-B_{12} in our blood because of our unique brains and circadian rhythm.

- If shellfish were not such a great supply of B_{12} and folate, all humans on earth would be speaking various Neanderthal dialects rather than a Homo sapiens language.

In sum, there is a deficiency of vitamers in our food, our supplements, and our bodies. Switching to B_{12} and folate in the bioactive forms can make a significant positive change in your health. They will help you defend against the internal and external challenges coming at you at an increasing rate.

We will now explore *The Vitamer Revolution*, the nexus of immune health (inflammatory response), epigenetics (environmentally influenced genetics) and vitamers (bioactive vitamins)—the science behind the future of your health.

Complexity

In writing this book, I am striving to explain a connection between three complex scientific domains: bioactive vitamins, epigenetics, and inflammation. There is so much factual material available from so many sources that I could not reference them all, so I am giving the known basics and my interpretation of them. I am not a genetic biochemist, but I have used my medical background to make these subjects more accessible for everyone. There will be some repetition of biochemical details and studies as they are important to fully understand the discussion of each subject at hand.

To the novice I will appear an expert, to the expert a novice. SZ

ONE

BUILDING A BETTER BRAIN WITH VITAMERS

Scavenged Meat→↑Brain Size→Hunting→↑Brain Size→
Stone Tools→↑Brain Size→Fire→↑Brain Size

Vitamins B12 and folate vitamers (collectively referred to in this book as B12/F) can truly be called the nutrients that created the human brain and thus, modern man. That's because the development of the brain was driven by increasing access to B12/F, which spurred the growth of larger numbers of brain cells and allowed the body to wrap each delicate nervous-system cell in a thick, protective myelin sheath, improving the ability of cells to form multiple connections with each other. Thanks to B12/F, our brains grew both larger and more complex.

Why was our small branch of the evolutionary tree, and ours alone, so fortunate? Why didn't tigers, who also consume large amounts of B12/F, develop advanced brains as well? Unfortunately, science has given us no clear answers. It may be that this is just the way evolution played out, driven by arbitrary forces such as climate change or the loss of a food source. Eminent scientist Stephen Jay Gould once explained the existence of humans by describing us as "*Homo sapiens*: a tiny twig on an improbable branch of a contingent limb on a fortunate tree." I guess we were just lucky. It's certain this luck depended on access to plentiful supplies of B12 and folate.

An Edible Complex

About four million years ago, our prehuman ancestors climbed down from the trees, became land-based omnivores, and began consuming a diet that included small mammals, reptiles, birds, and eggs. This gave them access to a richer concentration of nutrients I'll refer to as "meat," a simple label for the biologic complex of protein, vitamin B12, folate, iron, and fat found in animal tissue.

Prehumans mostly hunted for small animals that could be caught by hand, followed herds of larger animals in hopes of picking off strays, and fought with other scavengers for meat left behind by superior animal hunters. As they increased their access to meat, prehumans developed larger and more complex brains, making them better communicators and hunters. This, in turn, allowed them to access even more of the precious foodstuff, permitting their brains to advance further.

As their diets changed for the better with more B12 and folate vitamers from meat, the physicality of prehumans changed as well. Natural selection favored longer limbs, opposable thumbs, upright walking, and other characteristics we recognize today as being *hominid* (the primate family including humans and some of the great apes). To ensure a steady stream of B12 to the body's cells, the prehuman body developed a very specific, multistage, active transport system for this critical vitamer. Certain proteins bind B12 in the stomach as it is released from food. Other proteins transport it to the intestines, then carry it through the intestinal wall into the bloodstream, and finally deliver it to every single cell.

The prehuman body soon dispensed with the long intestine necessary for digestion of tough vegetable matter, for meat could be processed by a shorter digestive organ. This newly shortened gut had its downside, however. Besides being unable to digest highly fibrous foods like leaves, it couldn't synthesize certain vitamins and nutrients, such as vitamin C. None of this was a major concern millions of years ago, when our distant ancestors had easy access to the fruits, nuts, tubers, and other plant matter providing these nutrients.

It was at this point, 2.6 million years ago, that our ancient ancestors hit a wall and were unable to take the next evolutionary leap forward. Raw meat is tough to chew and digest, so there was a limit to how much they could consume and absorb. Lacking the power in their jaw muscles to break it down, they simply couldn't supply their brains with the additional nutrients required to advance further.

Then, some clever woman or man realized that certain kinds of rocks could be shaped into tools that could quickly cut meat into smaller pieces and pry the vitamer-rich marrow out of bones. These smaller pieces were much easier for stomach acid to break down, allowing prehumans to digest more meat. The new cutting tools also made it easier to scrape tiny pieces of raw meat off the bone so they, too, could be eaten. More nutrients than ever could be consumed before the meat went bad or was stolen by others.

Aided by this increased access to meat, our prehuman ancestors were able to stay alive, reproduce, and continue evolving better brains. Still, many groups lived on the edge of starvation or extinction. All it took was one season of drought, a few injuries, or a dwindling of the herd they followed to plunge them into serious danger. Then, about a million years ago, the cutting tool was transformed into a killing tool. It was simple: Just bang some rocks together in a progression of steps until a sharp point develops, put that pointed rock on the end of a stick, and you have a spear. Suddenly, prehumans could use their stabbing tools to bring down and butcher the animals they wanted to eat, and to fend off those who wanted to eat them. They could use the spears to drive scavengers away from freshly killed carcasses and protect themselves from other hominid marauders.

Brain development leaped ahead once again. Social communication skills improved, making it easier to plan and conduct hunts, defend the group, and cooperate with others in the raising of the young. Our ancestors rose even higher on the food chain, becoming top predators who could turn up their noses at picked-over, germ-laden carcasses in favor of the fresh meat they were able to provide for themselves. As their brains developed, so did their shoulder joints, allowing them to throw stones and spears with increasing accuracy and strength. They also mastered the craft of producing leather and fur clothing, which meant fewer calories spent protecting themselves from the cold. Every single calorie saved meant a better chance of surviving and more energy available to learn something new.

By this time meat could be cut into small pieces for easier eating, but it was still raw, difficult to digest, and a source of potentially fatal bacteria. Then someone came up with the brilliant idea of putting meat into a fire, perhaps by coming across animals that had been roasted in lightning-triggered savannah fires.

A Dedicated Taste for B12/F

Finding these nutritional gifts from the heavens solidified our craving for *umami*—the aroma and taste of cooked meat. Our mouths watered, then as now, when we smelled that smell and tasted that taste—our bodies knowing what we needed.

In 1903, Japanese scientist Dr. Kikunae Ikeda sought the source of that taste in protein by looking for the chemical causing it. What he discovered was that besides the four basic and well-known tastes of sweet, sour, bitter, and salty, we actually had an additional taste sensor, which he called *umami*. This word is derived from the Japanese word for "delicious," known as savoryness in English.

Umami was the only taste that developed for a particular kind of food. Because the protein/vitamer complex was so essential for growth, development, and fertility, our brainy ancestors developed a specific appetite for these crispy foods giving off such a unique aroma. They could track down those lightening-cooked steaks on the grasslands from miles away.

When Dr. Ikeda isolated the chemical responsible for umami, he also synthesized a stable artificial form that could be added to foods to provide some umami-like taste called monosodium glutamate (MSG). MSG is one way to add a savory flavor to vegetable dishes not having meat.

Frequent lightning-sparked fires provided high density protein-based vitamers on a predictable basis for a million years. By looking at a map of the surface of earth with the most number of lightning strikes, it is easy to see the most intense area occurs right over the savannahs of Africa where hominids developed. Whatever the source or inspiration, cooking meat made it much tastier, more sanitary, easier to chew, and easier to digest. That translated into a higher vitamer intake and a corresponding increase in brain size.

What Would We Do Without Fire?

To get some understanding of how hard it is to eat raw meat, take a brisket, chuck, or any tough cut of meat, grill it rare, and then try to rip off a piece with your teeth. Chew it, swallow it, then give your tired jaw muscles a much-needed rest. Now cut a small piece off, try again, and see if it is still a difficult grind. Being able to cut up the meat and cook it makes it a lot easier to chew and digest. Even with these advancements, it's still plenty of hard work and takes a lot of time. Welcome to your ancestors' world, and the reason for your wisdom teeth!

Once our ancestors mastered fire—yum, crunchy blackened BBQ!—they enjoyed a tremendous increase in calories consumed and could take in even more B12/F. They could also store cooked food for future consumption. This heat-sterilized meat may only have been safe to eat for a little while, but it was a tremendous improvement over raw meat, which attracts dangerous bacteria the minute it's exposed to air. Archeological evidence shows that, thanks to the development of tools and cooking about a million years ago, the size of the human brain increased by another third. Along with their bigger brains, our ancestors had fuller bellies, which meant they could spend less time hunting and gathering. This, in turn, gave them more free time to devote to teaching, the raising of offspring, and sex.

We've Been Burning Meat Forever

One of the oldest-known fireplaces, dating back more than 300,000 years, is located east of Tel Aviv in Israel inside an ancient limestone cavern known as Qesem Cave. This hearth was used by various Neanderthal and Homo sapiens families for millennia to warm themselves and cook their food, providing a captivating glimpse into humanity's remote past. This place would be a great location for a "Museum of Fire" and all that has derived from it. The next big discovery associated with fire was a fireproof and waterproof container that could boil heated liquids. "Now you're cookin'."

As evolution progressed, our ancestors became highly dependent on steady supplies of B12 and folate vitamers. By then they had taken on additional duties in the body, including controlling the hormones managing the immune response, a critical connection determining survival from life-threatening wounds and infections. B12/F also became vital for the production of pituitary hormones, facilitating and controlling pregnancy and loosening up the pelvic bones at the right time, enabling the increasingly large head of human babies to pass through the birth canal. Studies in fetomaternal medicine indicate the pituitary can increase in size by 50 percent or more during pregnancy, reflecting the massive increase in hormone production to support the fetus and thus a dramatic increase in the need for B vitamers.[5]

In ancient times, B12/F's role in fertility most likely served as a population control mechanism. When meat was plentiful, the consumption

---

[5] Dinč, F., "Pituitary Dimensions and Volume Measurements in Pregnancy and Post Partum: MR Assessment," *Acta Radiologica*, Vol. 39 issue: 1, January 1, 1998, 64–69.

of B12/F increased, leading to higher levels of pituitary sex hormones and increased fertility in both males and females. When a poor hunting season resulted in lower meat consumption, the levels of sex hormones, fertility, and births dropped.

A Mini-Ice Age, a Homo Sapiens Twig, Language Development, then Out of Africa

More than 100,000 years ago, a mini-ice age changed the climate just enough to dramatically alter the African landscape. Glaciers expanded around the world, soaking up water and significantly lowering the available atmospheric moisture. The resulting epic drought throughout Africa expanded the Saharan desert to such an extent the animal herds normally tracked out of Africa by humans died off. Imagine if the whole land area of the continental United States was a desert with only a narrow strip of land on the coast of Southern California able to support humans and small animals. Homo sapiens were now cut off from the rest of the world physically and genetically.

Neanderthals were also stressed and had to retreat from the expanding glaciers to southern Europe and southern Asia. During this retreat, the large-brained, heavily muscled, and spear-throwing Neanderthals wiped out all other Homo sapiens competitors north of the Sahara Desert.

Our ancestors were trapped in a hostile land of diminishing resources, and their numbers shrank. The scientific fields of paleontology, anthropology, geology, and ancient genomics all point to this one critical period in which only two thousand mating-pairs of Homo sapiens survived—our tiny twig from an improbable branch. Once this instance in time was defined, scientists had to find out where these Homo sapiens lived 70,000 years ago. To restate: *Everyone* on Earth is the offspring of these costal dwelling "Adam and Eve" couples.

Educated guesses led researchers to the southeast coast of Africa, where they focused on the exploration of coastal caves. Amazingly, they found DNA evidence—genomic fossils—of our progenitors in caves at Pinnacle Point and the Blombos Cave.[6] Besides finding their bones, an archeologic dig also found trash heaps, thereby discovering the basics of their diet of survival. The remnants revealed evidence of a carbohydrate-rich tuber (geophytes), small animal bones, and massive amounts of seashells. Evidently our ancient

---

[6] Marean, C., Bar-Matthews, M., Bernatchez, J. et al, Early Human Use of Marine Resources and Pigment in South Africa During the Middle Pleistocene," *Nature*, 2007; 449:905–908.

ancestors weathered the multi-millennial drought with this simple but nutrient-rich diet of carbs, protein, and vitamers to survive and thrive.

From Filter-Feeding to Bedroom Fun?

Oysters and clams contain high concentrations of B12 obtained from waterborne bacteria because they are filter feeders. Therefore, there may be some truth to the notion that eating oysters can stimulate sex-hormone production in B12-deficient pituitaries, acting as a mild aphrodisiac.

Climate Change, Vitamers, and the Origin of Language

Our ancestors survived by hunting the few surviving small game and gathering all the shellfish near the shore they could for the next three thousand generations. Isolation over time plus a steady source of vitamers set the foundation for Homo sapiens' greatest discovery, the most valuable survival tool in all of human history: language.

The enduring question of linguists around the world is: When and where did language develop? I will leave the definition of language to the scholars, but for the purpose of this discussion, language is the formation of a lasting set of words resistant to change to such an extent that it can persist in a large population and be consistently passed down over many generations. In other words, a language can be said to have developed when dialects have coalesced over time in one place long enough to become a permanent vocabulary throughout a larger population. Proto-linguistics, the science of early language, also points back to 70,000 years ago as a critical time in the development of Homo sapiens communication.

Before this time, all Homo species lived in small tribes with their own local dialects. These dialects lasted as long as the tribe did, before they were absorbed by others, migrated, or wiped out over time. This limited all kinds of knowledge and trade needed to be built upon generation over generation, such as tool production and birthing techniques. If a Neanderthal midwife in one tribe died, that knowledge died with her, putting her kinfolk at risk. Discoveries often had to be rediscovered over and over.

Alternatively, if a new medicinal herb or tool making technique was discovered and repeatedly conversed about by coastal Homo sapiens, their accumulated knowledge was expanded and improved upon generation over generation—*cumulative cultural evolution.* There is evidence near the coastal caves that our African ancestors learned how to use fire to transform certain rocks into microblades which were light enough to be eventually used as arrowheads.[7]

The bottleneck formed by the Sahara forced this population to talk to each other in their new language over and over again, becoming more defined as the millennia passed. Words and dialects coalesced into one predominant, shared, multigenerational language.

An Evolutionary Stable Strategy

Game theorists call a behavior, a gene, or any trait resisting outside influences an *evolutionary stable strategy*, a subset of the Nash Equilibrium. In the development of language, this occurs when a word is so ingrained in a population a new incoming competing word cannot be established.

It has been estimated that the last common ancestor of Homo neanderthalis and Homo sapiens lived over 600,000 years ago. Before the second Homo sapiens diaspora out of Africa, Neanderthals were the kings and queens of the world, having spread across a good portion of Europe and Asia. They had large brains, were evolutionarily bred to survive in a wide variety of environments, and they had the skills and tools to do so. They out-survived or wiped out almost all of the remaining hominid species, except for some Denisovans in Asia, until Homo sapiens reappeared. When our ancestors migrated out this time, we now had a language all Homo sapiens shared, and an arrowhead that when shot by a bow could kill at 100 feet, while spears thrown by Neanderthals were only effective at less than 50 feet. This made it relatively easy to kill the males and take their females.

The next significant innovation occurred 10,000 to 15,000 years ago: animal domestication.

Herd Instinct

No one knows quite how it started. Perhaps someone took a cute baby canine back to the camp for their child to play with. Maybe someone realized if an orphaned cow-like creature was confined to a small area, fed, and allowed to grow, it could provide enough meat for a great feast the following winter solstice. However it happened, humans learned to tame animals and breed

---

[7]Kyle S. Brown, et al, "Fire as an Engineering Tool of Early Modern Humans," *Science,*14 Aug 2009, Vol. 325, Issue 5942, pp. 859–862.

those who were the easiest to handle. The wild aurochs, for example, eventually became the domesticated cow, one of the few large animals that could be managed, fed, and mated with relative ease. The aurochs provided high-quality protein, B12, folate, and fat complexes, with a single animal yielding more than 1,000 pounds of meat. Aurochs became revered in those civilizations that domesticated it. This is noted in the Hebrew Bible where it refers to the worship of a golden calf, not a golden horse, golden goat, or golden chicken.

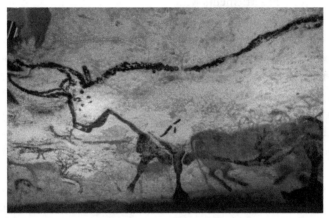

Cave Drawings of Wild Auroch

The downside to living in close proximity to a large number of domesticated animals is the cross-species infection by viruses, bacteria, and parasites continuing today. While it did stimulate the immune system, cross-species infection also introduced a significant health stress: the increased inflammatory response necessary for fighting off the assaults of new foreign pathogens. Inflammation is a necessary and healthy part of the immune response, but beyond a certain level, it is detrimental to health, and over time even potentially deadly. Manufacturing all the extra immune system cells required to handle cross-species infections also necessitated extra supplies of B12 and folate. (Much more about this later.)

In general, however, the domestication of animals was a giant leap forward for early humans conferring the advantage of somewhat more settled, seminomadic living. No longer required to follow the herds all year round, they could build semi-permanent settlements. By combining the meat obtained from domesticated animals and hunting with the vegetables, wild grains, fruits, and nuts gathered in foraging expeditions, people could generally count on a moderately steady supply of nutrients. Increased consumption of B_{12}/F improved fertility. Early humans still had to move from settlement to settlement when their animals overgrazed, or when all of the local fruits, vegetables and grains had been eaten.

Pita Wraps and Beer All Around

By 15,000 years ago, Homo sapiens had long developed modern brains and strong, healthy bodies, and they were skilled at making and using tools. They lived in small settlements with domesticated animals. They had battled through an evolutionary process that provided greater access to B_{12}/F, calories, and protein, stimulating greater brain development. This, in turn, translated into better protection against famine, harsh weather, infection, and so on. Yes, there were trade-offs, including a dependence on meat and exposure to new diseases, but all in all, humankind had benefited greatly.

Then something remarkable happened. Ten thousand to 15,000 years ago, humans began domesticating grains as a concentrated source of carbohydrate-based foods. In the Middle East, the grain was a new wheat hybrid; in Asia, rice; in the Americas (later on), it was maize. With calories and nutrients literally rising out of the ground, humans could feed themselves and their animals without being forced to move to greener pastures. Humanity leaped ahead on a new path that developed into the beginnings of the first cities, followed by city-states and empires.

Previously, slaughtering a single cow might provide a belly-filling meal for a hundred people or more. When grains were added to the meat, more than a thousand people could be fed. Toss in some vegetables, and the beef stew that resulted could be reheated many times without bacterial contamination. Thus, grains became the first "hamburger helper," making a limited protein source available to more people and allowing the local population to expand exponentially. Humans could use cattle to transport containers of grain when they migrated or marched as armies, then eat both the cattle and the grain, enjoying pita bread and beef kabobs any time they wanted. Once humans learned to store grain, they discovered that it sometimes spoiled delightfully to produce a parasite and bacterial-free alcoholic beverage called beer. For most of human history, beer has been a safer beverage than water.

Hoarding B12/Folate via Vampirism and Deification

Another life-altering effect of the domestication of animals was the opportunity to accumulate wealth in the form of livestock. As a result, socioeconomic classes began to emerge, spurring jealousy and anger, along with an increased need for some people to control others, if only to protect their nutrient wealth. Then there was the issue of managing that treasure: How does one get a nutrient infusion without unnecessarily sacrificing the expensive animals someone has worked so hard to acquire and fatten up? And how many domesticated animals can one afford to sacrifice to fill the bellies of one's extended family, while still retaining enough to breed and use for trade or dowries?

Every society has faced this dilemma, and each has come up with its own answers. In early Christian religions, days of fasting and weekly meat abstinence were integrated into daily life, reducing the slaughter of expensive animals. The Maasai tribe in Africa devised an elegant solution allowing them to save their cattle: Rather than a periodic slaughter of them for protein, they slit the cows' veins and drank their blood, making sure not to cut deeply enough, or drink richly enough, to kill the animal. This blood-snack was not as filling as a T-bone steak, but it did provide B12, protein, fat, and nutrients. This approach turned out to be quite successful, for until the introduction of "advanced" Western-style nutrition, the Maasai were a remarkably healthy, almost disease-free aboriginal society.

Hindu cultures preserved precious cattle by worshiping and caring for them. They collected the cows' milk over the course of many years of the animal's life. If they had slaughtered the cows just for meat instead and fed them to a starving population, they would have wiped out their herds and foregone an endless low-dose source of vitamers from milk products, as has happened in many other civilizations.

As populations increased and more land was devoted to grain production, there was a huge increase in available calories. This did *not*, however, increase B12 supplies, for there is no B12 in wheat, fruit, or vegetables. To make matters worse, meat was increasingly expensive, so less was consumed. As grains displaced B12 and folate in the diet, human health began to suffer. Today, in almost every part of the world, the disadvantages of a diminished intake of B12 and folate vitamers are widespread, something we'll discuss in the chapters to come. First, though, let's take a look at the history of the vitamers, beginning with B12.

TWO

THE DISCOVERY OF THE <u>VITAL</u> A<u>MINE</u>—B$_{12}$

Extrinsic Factor (Meat B$_{12}$)→
Ingestion + Intrinsic Factor (Stomach Protein)→B$_{12}$ Absorption

Since prehistoric times, healers have used various methods and substances to cure disease, both physical and emotional. Mothers, medicine men, midwives, and physicians paying house calls have all plied their patients with special foods and herbs, applied salves and creams, used hot and cold therapies, and administered hands-on healing techniques. Today's modern physicians examine patients with high-tech scans, scrutinize body fluids for minute amounts of telltale substances, prescribe pharmaceuticals, and perform surgeries. All of these methods, old and new, have some proven merit. No one ever thought there might be value in feeding, of all things, regurgitated food to patients—at least not until 1927. That's when Dr. William Bosworth Castle of Boston City Hospital used this bizarre method to treat patients suffering from pernicious anemia (the word *pernicious* meaning "insidious or deadly").

"Standard" low iron anemia is characterized by a shortage of healthy red blood cells and their constituent hemoglobin molecules, the function of which is to carry sufficient oxygen to all of the body's cells. Symptoms include weakness, fatigue, pale skin, and cold hands and feet. Pernicious anemia has the same symptoms, plus others: a sore and inflamed tongue, easy bruising, weight loss, gastrointestinal complaints, infections, numbness, depression, memory loss, and, in the latter stages, dementia and death.

Under a microscope, it's easy to see the difference between the two forms of anemia. Blood samples from patients with either standard or pernicious (megaloblastic) anemia show an abnormally low number of red blood cells. With megaloblastic anemia, however, the remaining red blood cells are overly large with immature, poorly developed inner structures indicating that they aren't making enough protein. These enlarged red blood cells are referred to as macrocytic or megaloblastic, which is why pernicious anemia is sometimes called *megaloblastic anemia.*

By the 1920s, healers knew that standard anemia could often be cured by feeding patients plenty of juicy red meat. Evidently an unknown "something" in the red meat was essential to the production of healthy red blood cells. Oddly enough, people with pernicious anemia did *not* respond to this treatment. Dr. Castle hypothesized there must be a *second* unidentified "something," manufactured by the body and necessary for utilization of the first unidentified "something" in the red meat. Those who were not cured by eating red meat, he theorized, must be missing this second, body-made substance. And the mystery substance might well be manufactured in the stomach, for autopsies showed that pernicious anemia patients had a greatly reduced number of gastric cells in the linings of their stomachs.

Given the limited experimental equipment available in 1927, Dr. Castle decided to test his theory in the most direct way possible. For the control part of the experiment, he gave his pernicious anemia patients the standard treatment: raw hamburger, delivered via a nasogastric tube inserted into the nose and passed through the throat into the stomach. As expected, this "meat infusion" did nothing to cure the illness. For the test part of the experiment, Castle himself ate raw hamburger and let it mix with his stomach juices for about an hour before forcing himself to regurgitate it. After the meat and stomach juice mixture had been allowed to incubate for a few hours, he passed it through a fine sieve, then infused the mixture into the patients' stomachs via a nasogastric tube.

After administering these treatments for several days, Castle took blood samples from the patients and examined them under a microscope. To his delight, he saw an elevation in the number of young healthy red blood cells, a sign of rapid red blood cell production. More importantly, his patients quickly recovered from what had typically been a fatal disease. Unfortunately, the novelty of his therapeutic process meant there was a limit to the number of patients Dr. Castle could treat—and the number of his dinner companions.

Castle's ingenious experiment proved that a healthy stomach (in this case his) provides a body-made substance that works with the "red meat substance" to treat pernicious anemia. He called the "red meat substance" *extrinsic factor* because it originated outside of the body, and the "body-made substance" *intrinsic factor* because it came from within the body. In 1948, studies performed by chemists Alexander Todd in England and Karl Folkers in the United States simultaneously identified the "anti-anemia factor" present in liver as vitamin B12. Seven years later, in 1955, researchers finally understood how the vitamin was structured. They gave it the scientific name *cobalamin* because it, unlike any other vitamin, contains a metal atom: cobalt.

The system for naming vitamins has had many authors and many detours from the first insights about them, categorizing vitamin A as fat-soluble and vitamin B as water-soluble. They found the B vitamin was actually different molecules working in similar ways, and they numbered them: B1, B2, B3, B5, B7, B9, B12. The naming system continued with the alphabet C to D to E to other letters. Many of those other lettered substances were dropped when the nutrients were found not to be vitamins. Ultimately, as Dr. Gerald Combs states in his textbook *The Vitamins*, previously referenced:

"... the accepted designation for the vitamins, in most cases, have relevance only to the history and chronology of their discovery, and not to their chemical or metabolic similarities."

In 1956, Dr. Dorothy Hodgkin, already a world-renowned x-ray crystallography expert, discovered the structure of B12. Her specialty was using x-rays to take pictures of molecules. By putting that information into a newly installed computer, she discovered the shape of B12 and that it contained over 180 atoms. For this discovery and all her other accomplishments, Hodgkin was awarded the 1964 Nobel Prize in chemistry.

Since then, medicine has learned that the mysterious intrinsic factor (IF), still referred to by this name, is a protein manufactured by cells in the stomach lining. Specifically, IF is a carrier protein that actively combines with and transports vitamin B12 and only B12 from the beginning of the small intestine to the end. There, the B12 is cleaved from IF and absorbed by the epithelial cells lining the intestinal wall, where it is attached to another carrier protein.

Pernicious anemia develops when the body doesn't get enough vitamin B12 to make healthy red blood cells, although this rarely results because of a lack of B12 in the diet. The problem develops usually due to autoimmune illness, alcohol abuse, medications, or infections that kill the cells lining the stomach that also manufacture IF.

A Complex Construction Job

While bacteria in the soil produces thousands of types of molecules, B12 is one of the most complex, requiring a thirty-stage biochemical construction process. Compare B12 to vitamin K, which is produced by intestinal bacteria. A molecule of vitamin K consists of three atoms of carbon, forty-six of hydrogen, and two of oxygen, for a total of fifty-one atoms. B12, on the other hand, requires sixty-three carbons, eighty-eight hydrogens, fourteen oxygens, fourteen nitrogens, one cobalt, and one phosphorus, for a total of 181 atoms. When finally assembled, B12 is more than three times larger and many times more complex than vitamin K; consequently, it is more vulnerable to chemical and environmental stressors impeding its bioavailability.

The following sections in this chapter and the next will provide some basic background biochemistry. Feel free to skip over as much as you want and come back to it at a later time when you have the overview down. It is not important to know all of this information, but it does supply a foundation to indicate how intricate this study can be if pursued further.

Four Forms of B12

As mentioned in chapter one, there are four substances referred to as vitamin B12 or, scientifically speaking, *cobalamin*. These four versions are identical except for a different attachment, or "arm," located at a specific place on the B12 molecule. While the differences between the four may seem insignificant—just one little "arm" on a large molecule—in the microscopic world of molecules, a tiny alteration in structure can make a huge difference in performance. These alterations give each version of B12 special properties. We live in an odd world where the most prevalent and least-expensive form of vitamin B12 happens to be the hardest one for the body to handle, even when correctly manufactured.

The first three forms are found only in soil bacteria. They start on their pathway when the soil is eaten along with the vegetation it is clinging to and takes up shop in the intestinal tract of ruminant animals. There they multiply, making additional M and A B12 forms.

Adenosylcobalamin (A-B12), a vitamer form of B12, is so-named because of

Vitamin B12

its adenosyl attachment. A-B12 makes up 70 percent of the B12 found in the body's cells, where it performs key functions. One of these is to act as a co-enzyme in the energy-producing process called the Krebs cycle. During the Krebs cycle, A-B12 assists in transforming a substance known as MMA into succinyl-CoA, aiding in the manufacture of the energy molecule adenosine-triphosphate, or ATP. ATP, sometimes called the "currency of the cells," is the energy molecule of most cellular processes, including DNA construction, red blood cell creation, and the healthy maintenance of nervous system cells. More A-B12 in the body translates into more circulating ATP, with cells better able to run at the high-energy levels necessary for reproduction, maintenance, and fighting off infection. When cellular energy levels crash, generalized fatigue and exhaustion result—adenosylcobalamin is the B12 of whole body energy.

Methylcobalamin (M-B12), one of two vitamer forms of B12, performs functions just as important as those belonging to A-B12. Named for its methyl group attachment (one carbon atom plus three hydrogen atoms), M-B12 is the vitamer form most commonly found in the human bloodstream at 70 percent, circulating until needed or converted by the cells into A-B12. Of the total cobalamin measured, the concentration of A-B12 is about 70 percent in the cells, with about 30 percent in the serum; M-B12 is about 30 percent in the cells and about 70 percent in the serum. This ratio is unique to humans, with all other animals having much lower percentages of M-B12 in their blood. M-B12 in the blood serves as a daylong resource converted into A-B12 as demanded by the needs of the metabolic cells.

Inside the cells, M-B12 and folate work together as coenzymes, detoxifying and converting a waste product called homocysteine into S-adenosyl methionine (SAMe). SAMe then helps control the expression/repression of numerous genes by functioning as a methyl donor for a DNA regulation process. When M-B12 is lacking, homocysteine is not converted into SAMe. Instead, homocysteine moves into the bloodstream, accumulating and exerting direct toxic effects on blood vessels in the heart and brain, increasing the risk of heart attacks, strokes, and dementia. Given the severity of these diseases, the importance of the cellular cleanup performed by M-B12 and folate cannot be overstated.

A lack of M-B12, vital for the production of red blood cell proteins, causes both general anemia and megaloblastic anemia. Increases in anxiety and depression are additional emotional health consequences of low B12. A certain type of antidepressants work by increasing the length of time neurotransmitters last in the synapse, the chemical communication space between nerve cells. If there is a deficiency of B12 vitamers (either M-B12 or A-B12), the manufacture of serotonin and other neurotransmitters cannot occur, and the response to antidepressants will be minimal.

Which Comes First?

It's interesting to note that in B12 deficiencies, the A-form has a much shorter half-life, so it runs out before the M-form. It is my interpretation that this is probably why the neurologic symptoms (numbness and tingling) linked to reduced A-B12 manifest before the red blood cell symptoms (megaloblastic anemia) linked to M-B12.

Why are humans the only animals with a preponderance of M-B12 vitamer in the blood? In all other animals, A-B12 is the predominant form in the blood. Why are we different? No one has ever established a reason, but if I were to hazard a scientific guess, I would say it's tied to our other human uniqueness, our large brains, which need a lot of nutrient support.

After a meal, the transporter protein for M-B12 lasts many hours longer than the transporter for A-B12, with the body quickly absorbing and distributing all of the available A-B12. This vitamer is integral to energy production, cellular metabolism, and repair mechanisms, which also generates waste products. M-B12, however, continues circulating in the blood throughout the day and into the night. During sleep our brain shrinks, allowing for an increased rhythmic flow of cerebrospinal fluid.[8] These pulsing currents of spinal fluid cleanse the cells of the waste product homocysteine and allow for the replenishment of neurotransmitters used up during the day. Circulating M-B12 along with folate converts the homocysteine into methionine. The M-B12 promotes myelination (insulation) of nerve cell axons and dendrites.

Hydroxocobalamin (H-B12), named for its hydroxyl attachment (an oxygen atom bonded to a hydrogen atom), is created by either soil bacteria or in the lab. Most of the H-B12 is converted by the animal's intestinal bacteria or the animal's liver into M-B12 or A-B12. Here in the United States, we use H-B12 for injections and oral supplements to a very modest extent, not nearly as much as do many other countries. H-B12 is also used for treating cases of cyanide poisoning, as cobalt has a powerful affinity for the cyanide molecule. When H-B12 is given to victims of cyanide poisoning, it donates its hydroxyl group in preference for a cyanide molecule, thus making cyanocobalamin (C-B12) in the blood. In other words, the basic molecule has such a strong preference for cyanide that it swaps out its hydroxyl group for cyanide, then safely tucks the poison within its structure, where it can no longer be of harm to you. That C-B12 can now be converted to M-B12 and A-B12.

Cyanocobalamin (C-B12) is essentially man-made and is the form of B12 found in most supplements and many medicinal injections. Back in 1948, when B12 was isolated and purified, the last step in the purification process was to put the liquid containing the B12 molecules through a charcoal filter. By some twist of fate, the charcoal contained an impurity, cyanide, that changed the natural versions of M-B12 and A-B12 into a synthetic form that was named cyanocobalamin. Cyanide conferred molecular stability to the vitamin and hence, a long shelf life, making it very economical to produce. For these reasons, C-B12 is now found in 99 percent of all supplements in the United States, and it is often the form injected into the body. However, before the body can utilize it, C-B12 must be converted through a multistep process into A-B12 or M-B12. The cyano-form easily combines with the vitamin C and/or iron found in supplements or food, becoming a macromolecule. This makes absorption by the body through the intestinal wall impossible. Thus, C-B12 is usually wasted when taken as part of a multivitamin.

---

[8]Nina E. Fultz, et al, "Coupled Electrophysiological, Hemodynamic, and Cerebrospinal Fluid Oscillations in Human Sleep," *Science*, November 1, 2019, Vol. 366, Issue 6465, pp. 628–631.

Can Sublingual Be Subtherapeutic?

Hoping to get C-B12 to the cells as quickly as possible, some people take a sublingual (under the tongue) supplement in an effort to maximize absorption rate and (theoretically) avoid having the nutrient routed to the liver. Paradoxically, this can actually slow utilization of C-B12, because it still needs to pass through the liver to be metabolized before it can be useful. Sublingual supplements simply dump C-B12 into the general circulation, where it must find its way to the liver to be converted to A-B12 or M-B12.

More problems arise once C-B12 arrives at the liver. Some people lack the enzymes—or sufficient amounts of these enzymes—to complete the process, because of liver damage or genetics. Or the liver may simply be too busy metabolizing alcohol, antibiotics, ulcer medicine, caffeine, birth control pills, hormones, or any of a wide variety of environmental toxins. In short, sublingual C-B12 *isn't* a faster route to the cells, and in some circumstances, it can actually be slower.

The important thing to remember about the four forms of B12 is that your body can only utilize the vitamin in the adenosyl or methyl forms—the vitamer forms. The cyano and hydroxyl forms must be converted before being used. When taken orally, A-B12 and M-B12 are absorbed quickly and reach all cells in the body. They also move into the brain to help maintain the nervous system, crossing the blood-brain barrier within thirty minutes of absorption. The vitamin forms, C-B12 and H-B12, cannot cross the blood-brain barrier until they are converted into the A or M forms. This is of critical importance since the brain needs these essential nutrients to function in an optimal way. It cannot do so unless the B12 molecules cross this barrier to support the brain just as glucose, proteins, and fats do.

There are many things you can do to increase your intake of B vitamers to improve your health, and other activities you can add to your toolbox to amplify their benefits. We will cover these in detail in future chapters.

Now that you know about the B12 molecule and how it is used in the body, let's see where it comes from.

The best overall reference book I have found for understanding the seriousness of B12 deficiency missed by the medical community was written by Sally Pacholok and Jeffrey Stuart: *Could It Be B12? An Epidemic of Misdiagnoses.* They clearly state the seriousness of this public health problem and how patients and their physicians are poorly prepared to address it. This essential book about an essential vitamin should be required reading in every medical school, as should this book.

THREE

B₁₂'s PATH FROM SOIL TO CELL

Bacterial B12→Meat B12→Human B12→Cellular B12→
↑Energy/Cell Maintenance

Vitamin B12 is unique among the vitamins in that it is produced only by soil bacteria. Plants don't manufacture or absorb this nutrient because they don't use it in their metabolic functions. Unlike vitamin D, created when sunlight comes in contact with the skin (photosynthesis), B12 is not manufactured by the body.

For the most part, bacteria produce B12 in the form of hydroxocobalamin (H-B12). Since plants have no use for B12, it is not absorbed, and it remains inside the bacteria in the soil or clinging to plant roots. There it sits quietly until an animal, let's say a cow, comes along and eats the tasty plant, along with a nice serving of bacteria-laden soil and perhaps a dash of animal dung, both of which typically contain B12 producing bacteria.

Bacteria surviving and reproducing in the cow's ruminal stomach move into the long loops of intestine, where they reproduce and create a lot more H-B12. This B12 finds its way into the animal's tissues, where it is converted into A-B12 and M-B12. These newly converted vitamers return to the bloodstream, where they are taken up by all of the cow's cells, especially those in the muscle tissue.

Once the cow has been processed and its muscle tissue converted into protein products such as hamburger, the two forms of B12 residing in the cow's muscle must survive freezing, storage, and cooking before finally arriving tucked inside a tasty morsel of meat on our plates. And once that meat is deposited into our mouths and we begin to chew, our bodies start the process of latching on to B12.

Just a Matter of Chyme

In the human mouth, the salivary glands churn out the first in a series of vitamer transporter proteins, called haptocorrin, that flow with the macerated meat into the stomach. Here, the stomach acids further break down the muscle tissue, releasing the B12 to combine with the haptocorrin. If you are over fifty, you might not be able to make enough acid to complete the breakdown, so your B levels could be low even if you have a normal dietary intake.

In brief, the B12/haptocorrin complex and the digesting liquid food (chyme) then moves along with IF (intrinsic factor) produced in the gastric cells, down into the small intestine. The B12 vitamers are cleaved off here by enzymes enabling the B12 to combine with IF. This remarkably complicated system is designed to protect fragile B12 along the route from mouth to cells.

As this IF/B12 macromolecule continues to flow down to the end of the small intestine, it is captured by special transport proteins units called cubam receptors on the intestinal cells (enterocytes). These receptors are responsible for transporting B12 into the cell. Another protein, multidrug resistance protein (MRP1), moves B12 from the cell out into the bloodstream.

Once inside the blood plasma, B12 attaches to another protein called transcobalamin. These TC/B12 complexes now flow throughout the bloodstream where they attach to every cell in the body.

This is a lot of saying hello and goodbye to partner proteins that take these vitamers from the mouth to the cells, but that's the means they need to take. A tiny bit of B12 does bypass this complex transport system and move into the bloodstream all by itself, via passive absorption. If it's not escorted (and protected) by a protein carrier, it's usually sent out of the body, unused, via the urine or bile within a short period of time.

As you can see, we humans have developed a very intricate system for absorbing B12. It's the only vitamin with such a complex, dedicated active-transport system for getting it to the cells. Why? There's a good reason: It's absolutely critical to our health!

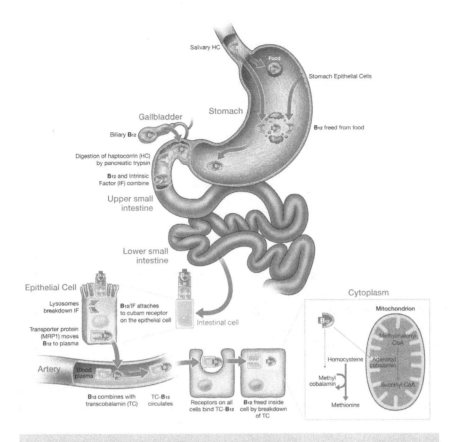

A Biochemical Tempest in a Teacup

While we absorb B12 from foods through an active transport system, we absorb most other vitamins—including the B12 we ingest via supplements—through a process called passive diffusion.[9] These vitamins pass through our intestinal walls "automatically," moving from an area of higher concentration to an area of lower concentration.

You can see an example of diffusion (passive transport) every time you put a tea bag into a cup of hot water. Soon after the bag enters the hot water, dark molecules from the tea leaves begin moving out of the bag and into the water. A standard *diffusion*

---

[9]You may recall mention of the passive absorption system for B12 in chapter one. While the body has developed active transport mechanisms for vitamers A-B12 and M-B12 from food, the C-B12 form found in supplements enters the body via passive transport in the intestines. Only 1 percent of C-B12 is absorbed this way, assuming the supplements are properly made and the passive absorption system is in good working order.

gradient with tea molecules moves from a higher concentration to a lower one. At first, the substances within the tea bag are highly concentrated, while none are present in the water. Over time as tea components leak out, the concentrations in both the tea bag and the water become roughly equal, and the process of diffusion is complete. An example of active transport would be if the tea bag could somehow pull the tea molecules *out* of the water and back into the bag.

Absorbing B12–Or Not

When A-B12 and M-B12 do not connect to their transporter proteins, they are urinated out within an hour or two. They must join these specialized proteins to last for longer periods of time in the blood. Otherwise cells won't have enough time to take up what they need to carry out their biochemical functions. The A-B12/TC complex remains intact for a much shorter time than the M-B12/TC complex, which can last many hours. This dynamic allows the M-B12 to be converted into A-B12 as needed over time.

Once the B12/TC complex arrives at the cell, proteins on the cell membrane grab it and pull it in. Before it can get to work, the B12 must be cleaved from its carrier protein. As you can see, the body expends quite a bit of energy identifying, separating, and protecting B12, and even more sending A-B12 and M-B12 straight to the cells while keeping some M-B12 at the ready in the bloodstream. Despite this, when all is working smoothly, A-B12 or M-B12 can arrive in the bloodstream and get into just about any cell in the body and cross the blood-brain barrier within about thirty minutes. If any cell needs extra A-B12, it has the additional option of snatching up some M-B12 and transforming it.

Unfortunately, this elegant system sometimes breaks down. Millions of people have difficulty with intestinal absorption and rely on sublingual B12 or B12 injections that bypass the passive diffusion of the intestinal route. If either supplement is in the form of C-B12, the benefits are diminished because cyanocobalamin must pass through the liver several times before being converted to bioactive A-B12 or M-B12. Few physicians or patients are aware of this; hence the continued use of less expensive and less efficient C-B12 sublingual or C-B12 IM forms. The fastest approach, and the one with the greatest bioavailability, would be an injection of A-B12 or M-B12.

Three Big Duties

You might think that because B12 is key to basic cellular metabolism, it must be directly involved in thousands of biochemical reactions. I certainly thought so when I began my studies. In truth, B12 is involved in two main tasks and one process: energy production and cellular cleanup along with the regulation of how genes are expressed. These biochemical reactions and their metabolic products are absolutely vital to the health of every single cell in the body.

(The next few sections contain some descriptions of biochemistry. It is not critical to know all these aspects to continue in the book other than to understand that A-B12 is critical for energy production, and M-B12 is critical for cellular cleanup.)

A-B12 and Energy Production

Energy the cell uses in biochemical reactions comes from a battery-molecule that stores one unit of cellular energy and is called adenosinetriphosphate (ATP). To get ATP energy you have to make it from succinyl-CoA but this requires A-B12. So, lack of A-B12 will translate into the reduced generation of cellular energy, leading to whole-body weakness, fatigue, and the "blahs." You can have a lot of C-B12 and even M-B12 circulating in your bloodstream, but if you don't have enough A-B12, in your cells they won't function at optimum efficiency.

It works like this: an enzyme breaks down various amino acids, fats, and cholesterol into a molecule called methylmalonyl acid (MMA), which is then converted, using A-B12, into succinyl-CoA. Next, succinyl CoA enters the energy producing Krebs cycle, generating power (ATP) that's used to run everything in the body. In short:

A-B12 + MMA→succinyl Co-A→Krebs cycle→↑energy(ATP)

In every biology and medical basic science course, there is almost always a review of the Krebs cycle at the beginning of the class. This energy producing cycle of the cell is so fundamental, elegant, and complex, it must be relearned many times. If you want to make a physician or biologist groan, ask them to explain the Krebs cycle.

When there's insufficient A-B12, methylmalonic acid (MMA) builds up in the blood. High levels of MMA damage the protective myelin sheath that covers the nerves. This is a main cause of the sensory neuropathy seen in B12/F deficiency. Without sufficient insulation, over time nerves' electrical signals become garbled, just like static on a bad cell phone connection. Loss of sensation, muscle control, and cognitive decline may result. A high concentration of methylmalonic acid (MMA) in the blood or urine is a telltale sign of poor vitamin B12 status.

The bottom line is, if you're lacking in A-B12, you may well be lacking in energy and have other problems related to deterioration of the myelin covers of the neurons of the nervous system. Numbness, weakness in the muscles, or the feeling of electric shocks under the skin are common symptoms.

M-B12 and Cellular Cleanup

Cleaning up waste products is an essential task, whether in the environment, your home, your body, or your cells. M-B12 vitamers play an important role tidying up the latter, especially when it comes to a molecule called homocysteine, which is toxic at higher blood levels.

Homocysteine is an amino acid produced by the body via a chain of biochemical reactions. It starts with methionine, an essential amino acid found in meat, seafood, eggs, and dairy products. In the liver, methionine is converted to a substance called S-adenosylmethionine (SAMe). SAMe is absolutely critical to the physical and emotional health of the body. Besides being a top-notch methyl donor, SAMe helps produce neurotransmitters like serotonin, dopamine, and epinephrine, all crucial to nervous system communication throughout the body. SAMe has a downside: once it has donated a methyl group, it becomes a different substance called homocysteine. Homocysteine is not your friend.

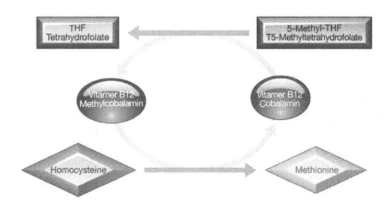

High homocysteine levels in the blood (a condition called hyperhomocysteinemia), damage the body's cells, particularly those lining the arteries. Resulting little wounds in the artery walls provide the perfect place for the buildup of plaque and clotting substances. High homocysteine levels also decrease the elasticity of the arteries, causing hardening of the arteries (atherogenesis), and increase the viscosity of the blood, causing blood clots (thrombogenesis). These negative factors raise blood pressure and accelerate the process of laying down cholesterol plaques in the heart, brain, and kidney arteries. Thus, it's not surprising that hyperhomocysteinemia has also been linked to an increased risk of heart attacks and strokes. Elevated plasma homocysteine levels are found in 5 to 10 percent of the general population, but in up to 40 percent of patients diagnosed with vascular disease.[10]

Further, homocysteine is a neurotoxin that interferes with the function of brain cells, making them more susceptible to damage and impairing communication between them. Some studies have shown an association between high levels of homocysteine and the onset of Alzheimer's disease and other dementias.[11] Hyperhomocysteinemia has also been linked to free-radical oxidation and aging, inflammation, a weakened immune system, and increased pain.[12] The excess of homocysteine has also been linked to oncogenesis: cancer production.[13] Fortunately, in a healthy body with enough B vitamers, homocysteine is reconverted into methionine or the body's strongest antioxidant, glutathione.

Charting the Steps

If we were to put B12's conversion of homocysteine into equation form, it would look like this:

M-B12/Folate/Methionine Synthase
↓
Homocysteine→Methionine→SAMe→↑Neurotransmitters/ DNA Modulation

---

[10] Stanger O, Herrmann W, Pietrzik K, et al, "Clinical Use and Rational Management of Homocysteine, Folic Acid, and B Vitamins in Cardiovascular and Thrombotic Diseases," *Z Kardiol*, June 2004; 93(6):439–53.

[11] David Smith, et al, "Homocysteine and Dementia: An International Consensus Statement," *J Alzheimers Dis.*, 2018; 62(2): 561–570.

[12] Henrieta Škovierová, et al, "The Molecular and Cellular Effect of Homocysteine Metabolism Imbalance on Human Health," *Int J Mol Sci.* 2016 Oct; 17(10):1733.

[13] LL Wu and JT Wu, "Hyperhomocysteinemia Is a Risk Factor for Cancer and a New Potential Tumor Marker," *Clinica Chimica Acta.*, 2002 Aug; 322(1-2):21–8.

In this equation, M-B12, folate, and the enzyme methionine synthase work together as enzymes, transforming the waste product homocysteine into the building block methionine. Without their enzyme action, the arrow leading from homocysteine to methionine would turn into a stop sign.

An active thinking brain creates a lot of metabolic waste that uses circulating M-B12 to reduce it back to methionine. The bulk of this chore is completed while you're asleep. M-B12 can last for hours in the bloodstream, continuing through the night, long after you've consumed that hamburger patty you had for dinner. While you're sleeping, M-B12 crosses the blood-brain barrier and gets to work maintaining your brain cells. You can think of M-B12 as the "clean-up vitamer," patiently floating throughout the bloodstream for hours, until needed.

The Process of Regulating Gene Expression

I said earlier that the B12 vitamers participate in only two major biochemical reactions: producing the succinyl-CoA needed for cellular energy and cleaning up homocysteine. But B12 is also essential to a process that literally changes the way your DNA behaves.

The B12 vitamers are necessary for *epigenetic methylation*, which is a way of modifying the "written-in-cement" expression of our DNA code. All it takes to help a "good" gene swing into action or to shut off a "bad" one is the attachment of a methyl group (one carbon atom attached to three hydrogen atoms). Epigenetic methylation is the same activity that determines whether an embryonic cell becomes a skin cell or a nerve cell, whether cancer genes are turned on or off, and whether our bodies respond to a stressor with an inflammation response that protects us or kills us. The methylation process, then, can literally make or break our health. We'll talk more about this in chapter five.

Love Your Liver

You can be sure that there is important biochemistry taking place in any body tissue containing a high level of B12. A case in point is the liver, which produces bile, blood proteins, and cholesterol, breaks down waste products, stores glucose as glycogen, regulates blood clotting, and metabolizes both toxins and medications. In most medical texts, the liver is incorrectly noted to contain a higher concentration of B12 than any other organ. These texts also assert that the liver stores several years' worth of B12. As a result, most physicians aren't alarmed when a patient isn't ingesting adequate amounts of B12, thinking there's plenty on tap in the liver. It is my belief (shared by various researchers in this field) that while our livers may contain plenty of B12, they do not store it for use in the rest of the body.[14]

In their research, Dr. LS Kornerup, et al., studied post-bariatric surgical patients (like Susan) finding:

> HoloTC and MMA were superior to B12 to detect early changes in B12 status following bariatric surgery. Our data challenge the current concept that liver B12 stores secure long-term maintenance of B12 status. They indicate that B12 treatment in pharmacological doses may be warranted immediately after surgery.

This means we may be at greater risk of B12 deficiency than previously believed.

Stores of B12 ≠ Stores B12—A Noun/Verb Misunderstanding

Many years ago, when researchers were trying to determine B12 levels in different parts of the body, the liver was described as having a large "store" of B12, meaning that it *contains* a lot. In my opinion, this was the result of a noun/verb confusion, transforming *stores* of B12 into *stores* B12. Storing suggests that the B12 is available for use by the rest of the body upon demand. In truth, vitamin B12 isn't "storable"—it's *water soluble* and can be easily urinated away. Storing B12 would require that it be kept in storage vesicles in the liver cells or attached to some special binding protein that could somehow last for years—but none of these things exists.

It's true that there is a lot of B12 contained in the liver, because the liver is a large organ. All of it is being used by the liver cells to perform their daily tasks. If the body uses this B12 for other purposes, the liver's ability to perform its own duties decreases. Think of it this way: There is the equivalent of many barrels of nails contained in the frame of a house, so you could say that the house has a large "store" of nails. If you start removing those nails for use elsewhere, your house will eventually fall apart.

---

[14] Kornerup L.S., et al, "Early Changes in Vitamin B12 Uptake and Biomarker Status Following Roux-En-Y Gastric Bypass and Sleeve Gastrectomy," *Clinical Nutrition*, February 15, 2018.

In my opinion, the liver earned its reputation for being a "B12 bank" when the total amount of B12 in the liver was first measured many years ago. The average liver contains about 2,000 micrograms of B12 in all its cells when the body is healthy, is supplied with plenty of B12-heavy foods such as red meat and shellfish, and has the ability to process it fully–in other words, the liver is in *luxus*. The body typically excretes about 2.4 micrograms of B12 per day, meaning that researchers calculated about one thousand days' worth of B12 residing in all the liver cells together—2.4 mcgs is the minimal daily requirement.

If you could take all of the B12 out of your liver and put it into vitamin pills, you could supply another person's daily requirements for a couple of years. How could the liver continue functioning at peak efficiency when it has "donated" much or all of its B12 content to the rest of the body? Even a 10 percent reduction in B12 levels in the liver would seriously hamper its function.

The critical point worth repeating is that most medical training and textbooks state that there is a three-year backup of B12 in the liver, and all *contemporary* healthcare is based on this incorrect assumption. Many medical treatments could be more effective if this B12 fallacy was corrected.

To make matters more complicated, the liver actually shrinks in both size and blood flow as it ages. By the age of sixty, the number of hepatic cells and the rate of blood flow through the liver have both declined by 50 percent, causing a decrease in liver function. The multistage conversion process required to turn C-B12 into vitamer B12 can be easily disrupted by aging or any stressor on the liver, such as infection or exposure to toxins. Alcohol use or certain medications such as proton-pump inhibitors, H-2 blockers, anti-epilepsy drugs, chemotherapy medications, SSRIs, anticoagulants, inhalants, and hormones like prednisone, estrogen, testosterone, and birth control pills reduce the body's use of B12 /F. Takeaway: Your liver is not a B12 bank!

The Mighty Liver

The liver controls more than 500 biochemical reactions producing new compounds and deactivating dangerous or foreign substances. The size of the liver gives an indication of its importance. To have evolved into such a large organ, it must have been very busy making proteins and detoxifying the poisons found in the carcasses and plants our ancestors routinely dined on. In modern times, the liver still needs to be sizeable in order to metabolize and detoxify the food and supplements we ingest, plus the environmental toxins we're constantly exposed to. We modern humans may live in a "safer" environment, but our ancient ancestors were never exposed to pesticides, polychlorinated biphenyls, xenoestrogens, and medications such as birth control pills, antibiotics, aspirin, acetaminophen, and more. Yet all of these must be metabolized, detoxified, and disposed of by our current one-and-only livers on a daily basis.

Pituitary Power

While the liver contains the largest amount of B12, it does not have the greatest *concentration* of B12 of all the organs, a misconception that can be found in most texts and references. The honor of the highest concentration belongs to the *pituitary gland*.[15] Per ounce of tissue, the amount of A-B12 and M-B12 in the pituitary is almost five times that found in the liver. Packed with so much B12, the pituitary is clearly "B12 Central."

Only one-fifth the weight of a penny, the pituitary manufactures critical hormones. These include follicle stimulating hormone (FSH) for egg and sperm production; luteinizing hormone (LH) to stimulate testosterone, progesterone, and estrogen production; growth hormone (GH) for growth and tissue repair; and melatonin stimulating hormone (MSH) to promote sun protection and to regulate sleep. B12/F is required to produce these hormones, which then travel through the bloodstream and balance the output of other hormone-producing glands in the body.

Another example of the B12/pituitary connection is seen in the thyroid gland. When signaled by the hypothalamus, the pituitary releases a hormone called thyroid stimulating hormone (TSH) that stimulates the thyroid gland to produce thyroid hormone. Too little TSH causes reduced hormone production from the thyroid, leading to hypothyroidism. So a sluggish thyroid can be due to a lack of TSH, thyroid hormone, and/or a lack of B12.

Not surprisingly, the symptoms of B12 deficiency are very similar to the symptoms of hypothyroidism: weakness, fatigue, weight gain, muscle pain, joint pain, brittle nails, thinning hair, memory difficulties, and depression. When people are given enough supplemental vitamer B12, among the first things they report are thicker nails and denser hair growth. That's because when there is enough B12 and folate to make thyroid hormone, optimum

---

[15] Cooperman, J., et al, "Distribution of Radioactive and Nonradioactive Vitamin B12 in the Dog," *Journal of Biological Chemistry*, 1960, Vol. 235, 191–194.

protein synthesis occurs throughout the body, the most visible being hair and nail growth.

Thyroid replacement hormone is one of the most common medications prescribed for individuals over fifty, the average age at which the body stops making enough stomach acid to extract sufficient amounts of B12 from meat. When doctors prescribe thyroid replacement hormone to treat hypothyroidism in someone with low B12, they might be ignoring the underlying problem. The patient could enjoy a short-term clinical improvement from the medication, but benefits will be limited because the body will still be deficient in *all* pituitary hormones. For all of the reasons discussed, it may be beneficial for patients treated for hypothyroidism to take vitamer B12 and folate supplements in addition to thyroid supplementation. (More on the B12/folate partnership in the next chapter.)

In short, supplying the body with adequate amounts of both A-B12 and M-B12 vitamers, as well as their metabolic partner folate, allows the pituitary and the areas influenced by its hormones to work at full efficiency. Conversely, anything that interferes with the bioavailability of B12/F, whether inside or outside the body, decreases the efficiency of every bodily function dependent on the pituitary—and there quite a few of these functions.

Sudden B12 Loss Is Nothing to Laugh At

It's an interesting thought-experiment to imagine what would happen to the body if B12 were depleted quickly rather than in the gradual manner usually seen in patients. Here's a real-life scenario.

It's no laughing matter, but the nitrous oxide used in dental procedures and general anesthesia blocks the body's ability to utilize any form of B12. Let's say you've been taking inefficient supplements, or you don't eat much food containing B12, or perhaps your body doesn't absorb nearly enough B12. Then you undergo a complex and lengthy surgery or dental procedure during which you inhale a lot of nitrous oxide.

Because nitrous oxide acts like a B12 blocker, once you're wheeled into recovery, you suddenly have much less B12 available for use than you should. After the surgery, you don't eat well due to discomfort and unpalatable hospital food, meaning you don't take in sufficient new B12 for wound repair and inflammation reduction. Suddenly you've got a significant B12 deficiency, manifesting in numerous ways, many of which will probably be overlooked by your doctor. Major postoperative complications, I suspect, may be due to a poor inflammatory and healing response caused by a lack of B12.

No B12 for NO2 Induced Deficiency

If the body stores three years' worth of B12, shouldn't the liver be able to donate its excess B12 to prevent such a sudden NO2 induced deficiency or return it to normal quickly? It doesn't because it can't.

There have been many case histories in which a patient goes in for back or hip surgery and is given nitrous oxide for anesthesia. The patients heal poorly due to reduced B12 and then have an episode of numbness and weakness of the legs, which is interpreted as another orthopedic problem. After a follow-up surgery with the use of nitrous oxide, the condition worsens. Someone finally looks at the blood, sees the macrocytic anemia, gets a B12 blood level measurement, and diagnoses subacute combined degeneration of the spinal cord due to a B12 deficiency. Injections are ordered too late, and the nerve damage cannot be completely reversed.

B12 deficiency spinal damage has also been documented from the recreational use of whippets—whipped-cream NO2 dispensers.[16]

These case histories underscore the vital point that by the time clinical symptoms of sensory nerve damage show up, it's been around for a while and might already be irreversible.

The graphic below gives many of the dietary sources of B12 to be explored.

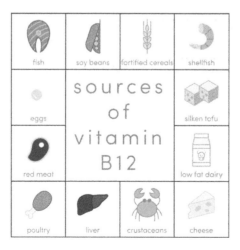

---

[16] MDuque, Miriam, et al. "Nitrous Oxide Abuse and Vitamin B12 Action in a 20-Year-Old Woman: A Case Report," *LabMedicine*, 46, 2015, 312–315.

In a Nutshell

As I'm sure you'll agree, the route B_{12} takes from soil bacteria to the cells of the human body is intricate and fraught with danger. It takes just a single genetic abnormality, a minor metabolic complication, a medication side-effect, a poorly made supplement, or some other difficulty to bring this journey to a screeching halt.

B_{12} and folate are obligatory co-factors requiring adequate levels of each to function optimally in maintaining cellular homeostasis. The form and function of folate is the next exploration.

FOUR

FOLATE, THE "PARTNER VITAMER"

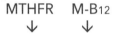

MTHFR   M-B12
  ↓   ↓

Folic Acid→Folate→↓Homocysteine→↑Methionine→
↑DNA Methylation→↓Birth Defects

The vitamin known as folate (B9) is B12's "partner vitamer," with the two nutrients working in tandem to keep the body energized and functioning at high capacity. The word *folate* is often used as a catchall term referring to all members of the B9 group, but here I am using it to identify the active vitamer form. And while "folate" and "folic acid" are often conflated by the medical, research, and manufacturing communities, there are vital differences between them:

- *Folate is scientifically known as 5-L-methyltetrahydrofolate (5-MTHF) or L-methylfolate.* These are the names of the natural B9 vitamer, the *final* biochemical form of B9 that the body utilizes. Folate is also the only form that can cross the blood-brain barrier and make its way into the brain, where it performs important clean-up duties. Confusingly, the term *folate* is sometimes used as an umbrella word for multiple vitamin forms that may be eventually metabolized by the body into folate. For example, folic acid is often confused with folate. Pre-vitamer forms of folate are found in many common plant foods, including spinach foliage. The word *folate* is derived from the word *foliage*. Higher concentrations of the vitamer folate present in liver, egg yolk, beef, chicken, and are more easily absorbed by the human body from these sources. Bioavailability of folate from these foods depends on many factors, the first being how the food is processed, stored, and prepared. The vitamer folate is sensitive to heat, light, and certain foods which can inactivate it. This is why vitamers should always be taken with water and not juice or food. Ironically, folate cannot work well without enough vitamin C and iron in the body, but they should not be ingested together.

Folate works with B12 to generate energy and cleanse the cells of waste, aids in the manufacture of new cells, promotes fertility, and protects against alterations in the expression of DNA that might result in cancer. It also plays a role in:

- Production of immune cells to fight viruses, bacteria, and cancer
- Synthesis of brain chemicals related to mood, appetite, sleep, and short-term memory
- Inflammation control
- Repair of nerve cell membranes
- Heavy metal detoxification
- Production of glutathione, which is the body's strongest antioxidant
- Red blood cell development, DNA synthesis, protein formation, and fat metabolism

Medical conditions increasing the body's need for folate include gastrointestinal malabsorption syndromes, pregnancy, excessive physical exertion, and most serious medical illnesses. Symptoms of a folate deficiency include anemia, weakness, lethargy, gray hair, mouth sores, and growth problems. Too little folate has been linked to neural tube defects in unborn children, as well as cancer, heart disease, depression, and other medical problems.

If you are fortunate, your body absorbs an average of about 50 percent of the folate in your food, although the amount varies from 10 to 90 percent depending on the food, its freshness, and how it is processed, stored, and prepared. Since folate is sensitive to heat, light, oxygen, and contact with other foods, much of it disappears during cooking or processing, and when it's exposed to the air. Quick-frozen or freshly harvested vegetables, and fresh, lightly cooked meats are the best sources of this vitamer.

- *Folic acid is the synthetic form of folate used in food fortification and dietary supplements.* Folic acid cannot cross the blood-brain barrier but, like C-B12, folic acid is more stable than the vitamer form folate. This gives folic acid a longer shelf life and explains its use in fortifying enriched grain products including bread, flour, cornmeal, rice, and pasta. The downside is that the body must convert the artificial folic acid into folate before the vitamin can be used. If it isn't converted, the folic acid just floats uselessly—though not necessarily harmlessly—through the bloodstream until it's eliminated.

Because of limited inheritance of the right kind of genes, the conversion process is genetically impaired in more than 50 percent of the population; therefore, many people don't use sufficient amounts of folate even though they're consuming large amounts of folic acid via fortified foods and vitamin pills. If they can't convert well, people won't have enough folate to work as a co-enzyme with B12. This means they don't generate enough cellular energy to sweep away cellular waste, which means . . . well, you get the picture.

- *Folacin is another rare form of B9 you may have seen on a few supplement bottle labels or in research papers about folate.* Folacin is "in-between" folic acid and folate and must still go through two more conversion steps to become the vitamer folate. It is sometime referred to as folate on supplement labels, but it is not.

What Causes Folate Deficiency?

There are several reasons why you might find yourself lacking in folate. You may consume inadequate amounts via your diet, or your body might absorb the vitamin poorly. People who overuse alcohol can develop a deficiency because an abundance of folate and other B vitamins are required to metabolize alcohol. Alcohol abuse coincides with poor nutrition and poor folate intake. Conditions like celiac disease and interactions with certain drugs, including anticonvulsant medicines and oral contraceptives, cause reduced folate blood levels. Other medications, such as metformin and methotrexate, also deplete folate. Folate deficiencies may also occur during times of increased need for the vitamin, including infancy, pregnancy, lactation, or illness. The most common, least recognized cause of deficiency is obesity since adipose tissue requires a lot of folate for its self-maintenance.

Two additional factors limit vitamer conversion of folic acid in food and supplements into methylfolate. As you will see below, four steps are involved in the full transition of folic acid into folate. The last step uses the MTHF reductase (MTHFR) enzyme to finalize the production of folate. Certain medications limit the effectiveness of this crucial enzyme.

The other common reason people have a folate vitamer deficiency is a genetic code mutation that limits or entirely prevents the transformation of folic acid into folate because these folks don't make enough MTHFR enzyme. There are actually more than thirty different mutations that change the shape of the enzyme (polymorphisms) and prevent it from working. The most common is a cytosine-to-thymine mutation at the 677 locus on your gene called a *C677T MTHFR polymorphism mutation*. If one gene doesn't work with a C677T mutation, the normal gene C677 on the other chromosome can work, but with an overall decreased folic acid-to-folate conversion. It is estimated that 50 percent of people have one good gene and one bad (heterozygous). When there is a mutation with two C677T genes (homozygous), found in 25 percent of people, the lack of the MTHFR enzyme is a significant deficiency. These unfortunate individuals are at risk for every illness caused or worsened by low folate—cancer, dementia, diabetes, etc.[17,18,19]

The "Last Vitamin"—How Folate Was Discovered

During the twentieth century, as one vitamin after another was identified and isolated, the substance called folate emerged as one of the last revelations. Its discovery began in the late 1920s when Dr. Lucy Wills journeyed to India multiple times to study pregnant women suffering from macrocytic anemia. After much observation, Dr. Wills hypothesized a connection between anemia and the women's diets. She began experimenting with monkeys until she reproduced the anemia. When she discovered a yeast extract that relieved symptoms in the monkeys, she knew she was on to something. However, another ten years would pass before the substance in yeast was identified as a vitamin and labeled folate. The name reflected the tons of

---

[17] Susanna C., et al, "Folate Intake, *MTHFR* Polymorphisms, and Risk of Esophageal, Gastric, and Pancreatic Cancer: A Meta-analysis," *Gastroenterology*, Volume 131, Issue 4, October 2006, 1271–1283.

[18] Cajavilca, C, et al. "MTHFR Gene Mutations Correlate with White Matter Disease Burden and Predict Cerebrovascular Disease and Dementia," *Brain Science,* 2019, 9(9), 211.

[19] Yanzi Meng, et al, "Association of *MTHFR* C677T Polymorphism and Type 2 Diabetes Mellitus (T2DM) Susceptibility," *Molecular Genetics & Genomic Medicine*, 30 October 2019.

foliage (spinach leaves) researchers were forced to process in order to isolate and identify folate.

This new cure was unfortunately difficult to administer, because the vital vitamer began "falling apart" soon after extraction, not lasting long enough to be administered to patients. Finally, in 1943, a man-made stable form of the vitamin with a long shelf life was developed and given the name folic acid. Doctors continued to pay little attention to folate deficiencies because no one really knew what a lack of the vitamin did to the human body. Toward the end of the 1950s, Dr. Victor Herbert noticed that one of his anemia patients responded quickly when he gave him low-dose folate supplements. This patient had long been consuming a strange and limited diet of doughnuts, steamed hamburgers, and coffee, giving Dr. Herbert an idea for an experiment to see what happened when one deliberately ate a folate-deficient diet. All he needed was a volunteer who would consume a folate-free and possibly life-threatening diet for about five months. Finding no volunteers, Dr. Herbert volunteered himself.

For his study, Dr. Herbert only consumed food that had been boiled three times, knowing all that soggy cooking would inactivate folate. Soon enough he developed the classic symptoms of folate deficiency: weakness, lethargy, constant fatigue, irritability, depression, and a sore tongue. A microscopic look at his red blood cells revealed he was suffering from macrocytic anemia.

Dr. Herbert's groundbreaking study led to further research linking folate deficiency and nerve damage, depression, and dementia. Folate deficiency was eventually declared a public health crisis, resulting in the passing of a 1998 U.S. law requiring that folic acid be added to bread and other grain products to ensure sufficient amounts of this important vitamin for the general public.

The significance of this public health intervention is on par with the law requiring polio vaccinations. This folic acid supplementation law reduced spinal cord birth defects by 85 percent.

How Folate Works to Keep You Healthy

Methylfolate plays several roles in cellular metabolism, the two most important of which are cleansing the cells of homocysteine and regulating DNA expression of healthy genes.

When the agouti gene mice received sufficient folate, they had healthy bodies and body weight, and had a much lower incidence of heart disease, diabetes, obesity, and premature death.

The Agouti Gene

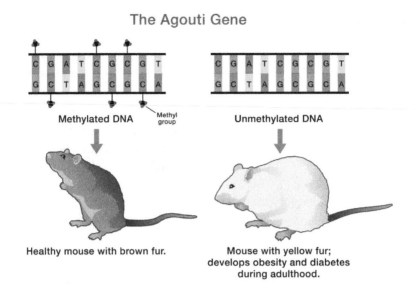

Methylated DNA — Methyl group   Unmethylated DNA

Healthy mouse with brown fur.   Mouse with yellow fur; develops obesity and diabetes during adulthood.

Toxic Trash–Getting Rid of Excess Homocysteine

As stated earlier, M-B12 and M-folate work as a team to clear the blood of excessive homocysteine by converting it into a substance called SAMe. SAMe has several important uses in the body, including production of DNA and RNA, maintenance of cell membranes, and manufacture and breakdown of neurotransmitters. If either vitamer folate or B12 is in short supply, excess cellular homocysteine doesn't convert into SAMe, and the homocysteine levels rise. This leads to hyperhomocysteinemia, which drives up the risk of autism, developmental delays, heart disease, strokes, cancer, depression, and dementia.[20, 21, 22]

[20] Zablow, S., "Folate Deficiency Based Autism as an Orofacial Clefts/Neural Tube Defect Spectrum Disorder," *JAACAP*, November Issue 11, 1126–1127, Vol. 58, 2019.
[21] Zablow, S., "Reader Response: Hemoglobin and Anemia in Relation to Dementia Risk and Accompanying Changes on Brain MRI, *Neurology*, August 15, 2019 (online).
[22] Larsson, S. C., "Homocysteine and Small Vessel Stroke: A Mendelian Randomization Analysis," *Annals of Neurology*, February 19, 2019.

Deciphering the Homocysteine Riddle

Lack of folate and B12 are linked to a buildup of homocysteine. The danger posed by elevated homocysteine was discovered– or more precisely, stumbled upon–by Dr. Kilmer McCully at Harvard Medical School in the late 1960s. As part of his regular duties, Dr. McCully was reviewing the autopsies of children who had died of a rare genetic blood disorder that caused hyperhomocysteinemia. He noticed the children were all felled by medical conditions usually seen in the elderly, such as hardening of the arteries, heart attacks, strokes, and blood clots. What, he wondered, was the link between homocysteine and the way-too-early onset of fatal cardiovascular disease in these children? The hypothesis he developed was profound: Excess homocysteine must be a powerful risk factor for cardiovascular disease, perhaps even more harmful than elevated cholesterol.

Dr. McCully theorized that excess homocysteine weakens cells lining the inside of blood vessels. As a result, their collagen walls and collagen connections to each other begin to falter. The body responds by making cholesterol/collagen patches that become part of the cell wall and, in the process, undermine it. That is, the patch solves the immediate problem but continues to grow bigger and thicker, eventually pushing its way into the bloodstream, where it interferes with the flow of blood. Even mildly elevated homocysteine, then, could be a significant contributor to cardiovascular disease.

As Dr. McCully worked to piece this puzzle together, powerful forces began to work against him. His colleagues balked. They wanted him to only look at the elevated cholesterol theory of atherosclerosis, the "big thing" at the time, and figure out how to fight heart disease with cholesterol-lowering drugs. By challenging the accepted wisdom, Dr. McCully was threatening to debunk the theory that paid the bills for so many of his colleagues. Perhaps worst of all, he proposed treating the condition with relatively inexpensive B-vitamins instead of the pricey medicines produced by the pharmaceutical companies supporting so much of the research.

In response, the medical and research communities turned their backs on McCully, costing him his job and professional reputation. In the 1990s, when the results of clinical studies began supporting his theory, McCully was vindicated. More than thirty years after first coming up with his hypothesis, medical researchers finally accepted the idea that cholesterol wasn't the only villain in town. Excess homocysteine was also deemed a powerful risk factor for cardiovascular disease. Ironically, it was a study of 14,000 physicians—including some who had doubted and denied Dr. McCully—that showed a high blood level of homocysteine increases the risk of cardiovascular disease.[23]

Preventing Neural Tube Defects

As the developing embryo grows into a fetus, DNA expression leads cells to differentiate into three distinct layers. The first, the endoderm, develops into the gastrointestinal, respiratory, endocrine, and urinary organs. The second, the mesoderm, becomes muscle, bone, fat cells, and cartilage, while the third, the ectoderm, develops cells that differentiate into skin, hair, nails, brain, and nerves. (Interestingly, all tissue cells deriving from the same layer "talk" to each other through protein messengers for the rest of a human's life—i.e., fat cells closely communicate with muscle cells.)

The three layers of cells—endothelial, mesothelial, and ectothelial—fold around each other, guided by B12/folate-controlled DNA methylation that carefully times the expression of the genes. At the proper point in time, the ectoderm folds itself into a tube, with skin cells on the outside and nerve and spinal cord cells on the inside. This tube eventually squeezes itself closed and becomes the neural tube housing the brain and spinal cord. This complicated series of events must be perfectly coordinated if the future baby is to have a normal nervous system.

A neural tube defect occurs when the tube does not completely envelop the brain or spinal cord to seal shut, resulting in devastating conditions including spina bifida and brain malformations such as anencephaly and hydro-anencephaly.

Warding Off Unrecognized Neural Tube Defects?

Pilonidal cysts are infection-prone fluid-filled sacs at the base of the spine.

---

[23] Ubbink, J.B., "Vitamin Nutrition Status and Homocysteine: An Atherogenic Risk Factor," *Nutrition Review*, November 1994, 52(11):383–7.

Studies have shown that there is a powerful association between the risk of developing pilonidal cysts and having a mother who took medications blocking the conversion of folic acid into folate during her pregnancy. These meds include ondansetron, lansoprazole, lamotrigine, nitrofurantoin, and valproic acid.

Might there be more? Could neural tube defects (NTDs) exist on a continuum, a spectrum, rather than as a series of discrete diseases? The greater the stressor (i.e., low maternal folate), the more severe the defect. If this trail of neurologic consequences is followed toward one end of the folate-deficiency disorder spectrum, might we discover some forms of autism and other developmental disorders belonging in that range? After all, there is a higher incidence of autism in children born to folate-deficient mothers.[24] Can this thinking extend even further? Is it possible that a propensity toward post-traumatic stress disorder (PTSD), depression, autism, and attention deficit hyperactivity disorder (ADHD) belong on this spectrum, as seen in the diagram below?

Prenatal Folate Deficiency; Neural-Tube Defect Spectrum

	Upper NTDs	Lower NTDs
Severe folate deficiency →	anencephaly	spina bifida
↓	↓	↓
Moderate folate deficiency →	hydro-anencephaly	spina bifida myelomeningocele
↓	↓	↓
↓	cleft palate/ cleft lip	pilonidal cyst
↓	↓	↓
Mild folate deficiency →	autism, PTSD, depression, anxiety	spina bifida occulta

---

[24] Gao Y, Sheng C, Xie R-h, Sun W, Asztalos E, Moddemann D, et al, (2016) "New Perspective on Impact of Folic Acid Supplementation during Pregnancy on Neurodevelopment/Autism in the Offspring Children—A Systematic Review," *PLoS ONE* 11(11): e0165626.

At this point, no one knows for sure. What is known is that a lack of folate is linked to some serious nervous system disorders, some moderately serious ones, and some that only show up on random x-rays. Should science stop here, proclaiming the absolute limits of folate-nervous system relationship? Hardly. The case is not closed.

A Misguided Approach?

Just before the dawn of the twenty-first century, the United States government mandated that certain foods be fortified with folic acid, a well-intentioned effort to ward off neural tube defects in unborn children whose pregnant mothers have low folate levels.

By anyone's standards this program was a resounding success, reducing the incidence of NTDs by as much as 85 percent in some studies. Still, why not aim higher? What about the 15 percent of fetuses who developed folate-deficiency-driven NTDs despite grain fortification and vitamin supplementation? I believe many of these mothers-to-be were genetically unable to metabolize folic acid because they lacked the "conversion enzyme" MTHFR necessary for folate metabolism. Taking the artificial folic acid form of the vitamin did them no good. If they had taken the vitamer form of folate, the results for some would have been far better. I firmly believe that a lab test for MTHFR status should be performed on every woman wishing to become pregnant in order to discover whether she can transform folic acid into the vitamer folate. One day soon this potentially lifesaving and inexpensive blood test will become routine.

Metabolizing Folate, Both Natural and Artificial Forms

Like B12, most folate resides in the liver where it is used (not stored) by every hepatic cell. The bioavailability of folate from a variety of foods varies widely. The way the body handles the vitamer folate differs in important ways from how it handles artificial folic acid. The pre-folate forms found in food can be converted into folate (5-methyl-tetrahydrofolate) in the intestines and undergo active transport into the blood. Folic acid is only absorbed by passive diffusion.

To clarify the confusion about the different forms of B9 found in foods, dietary folate equivalents (DFEs) were established. DFEs denote the greater absorption of folic acid compared to food folate. One microgram (mcg) of food folate equals 0.6 mcg of folic acid, just as one microgram of folic acid equals 1.7 mcg of food folate. The standard minimal intake of folate recommended is 400 mcg per day (400 mcg DFEs) or 240 mcg of folic acid (400 mcg DFEs), assuming the body can absorb the form of folic acid provided and can convert the folic acid into the vitamer folate and a woman is not pregnant (which requires more). In a later chapter, I suggest an optimal intake.

The following graphic identifies some good dietary sources of folate.

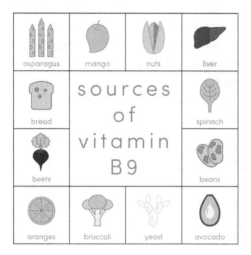

How does this happen? Let's start by looking at the folate vitamer, the form your body was designed to utilize. Imagine you've just taken a bite of spinach, chewed it well, releasing folate and a wide variety of folate precursors from the fiber, and swallowed it. The salad greens you ate travel to your small intestine, where some of the folate it contains attaches to special receptors in the intestinal cells. From here, the vitamers of folate are free to be absorbed directly by the cells of the body and brain.

(What follows is some biochemistry that you can skim. The important point here is that if you don't have the MTHFR enzyme or enough folate, your life is not going to be so pleasant.)

Folate precursor forms are transported to the liver, where vitamin B_{12} plus an enzyme called MTHFR (methyltetrahydrofolate reductase) convert it into its active form, 5-methyl THF—the vitamer. If any of the elements (M-folate, MTHFR, or vitamin B_{12}) are missing, this process will not take place. Here's the progression, in two equations:

$$\text{MTHFR} + \text{B}_{12}$$
$$\downarrow$$
$$\text{Dietary Intake} \rightarrow \text{Tetrahydrofolate (THF)} \rightarrow \text{5-methyl THF}$$

$$\text{B}_{12}$$
$$\downarrow$$
$$\text{5-methyl THF} + \text{Homocysteine} \rightarrow \text{Methionine} \rightarrow \text{SAMe} \rightarrow \text{DNA Methylation}$$

Transforming folic acid from a supplement or fortified grains into SAMe is a more complex procedure than the one we just examined. Like other folate precursors, the man-made folic acid makes its way through the small intestine and into the liver. Once there, it must go through a four-step process that requires the enzyme *dihydrofolate reductase* to transform it into tetrahydrofolate (THF). Only when it's been transformed into THF can it be converted by MTHFR into the active vitamer form, 5-methyl THF.

This diagram shows the necessary complex steps to covert folic acid or dietary folate precursors to the vitamer folate, with the MTHFR enzyme participating in the final step.

$$\text{Supplements/ Fortified Food (Folic Acid)} \rightarrow \text{DHF} \leftarrow \text{Diet (Folate Precursors)}$$
$$\downarrow \quad \leftarrow \quad \text{DHF Reductase}$$
$$\text{THF}$$
$$\downarrow$$
$$\text{5,10 methylene- THF}$$
$$\downarrow \quad \leftarrow \text{MTHF Reductase}$$
$$\text{M-Folate - the vitamer}$$

Dihydrofolate reductase is not terribly energetic and active; therefore, it is not efficient at transforming folic acid into folate. Thus, lots of unmetabolized and unusable folic acid ends up floating around in the bloodstream, even after ingesting as little as 200 mcg. That's just not good. Too much folic acid in the blood gums up the works, possibly reducing the flow of folate across the blood-brain barrier. Blocking the flow of the folate into the brain deprives the brain of the tools it uses to do its work of cleansing and cell maintenance.

The Importance of MTHFR

Folic acid is metabolized poorly by people who have inefficient MTHFR. For these folks, folic acid supplementation will be about as helpful as giving a wax apple to a starving person and will put them at risk of every illness caused or worsened by low folate. A sampling of disorders related to mutations in the MTHFR mechanism includes: Alzheimer's disease, high homocysteine, multiple sclerosis, recurrent miscarriages, increased risk of having a baby with neural tube defects, depression, diabetes, stroke, many kinds of cancer, epilepsy, and childhood learning disorders.

Even in those who don't have a MTHFR mutation, the enzyme's action can be blocked by anticonvulsants such as phenytoin and primidone; the diabetes medication metformin, the ulcerative colitis medication sulfasalazine, and barbiturates, to name several.

Massive Misdiagnosis?

Low folate levels have been associated with a poor response to antidepressants, forgetfulness, difficulty concentrating, irritability, depression, behavioral changes, and memory loss. A shortfall of B12 and other nutrients has also been tied to mental and emotional distress, as well as problems with nerves, muscles, and balance. Since medical professionals rarely consider potential vitamin deficiencies, some people with low levels of B12/folate have been erroneously treated for multiple sclerosis, Alzheimer's disease, fibromyalgia, Parkinson's disease, dementia, and depression, while their B12/F deficiencies are missed entirely. So much suffering could be avoided if these deficiencies were tested in patients before other more expensive and invasive tests are ordered. Folate and B12 could then substitute for or augment otherwise sub-effective therapies.

Remember the agouti mice? The yellow obese mice died sooner because of their folate-deficient diet. In the next chapter, we'll review DNA epigenetics to explain the vitamer-deficiency mechanism damaging the cells and leading to increased inflammation.

FIVE

NUTRITIONAL EPIGENETICS: YOU ARE WHAT YOUR GRANDPARENTS ATE

↓Folate→↓Methylation→
↓Agouti Gene Suppression (↑expression)→↑Illness

Have you been told you have your father's hands or your mother's eyes? That your chin dimple was passed down to you by your grandfather? These characteristics are most likely part of your genetic legacy, the sum total of the genes you received at conception. For the rest of your life, your unique genes will determine what you look like, how things work inside of you, how you age, and more.

Your genes are composed of a substance called DNA (deoxyribonucleic acid). DNA contains the "instructions" needed to create almost every protein in your body. Proteins give your body its structure and are crucial for the processes that keep it working and in a healthy balance. From conception on, your genes are "carved in stone," so to speak; they are not supposed to change. (If they do, you've got a genetic mutation that could cause a lot of trouble.) In many cases, however, there are mechanisms modifying the expression of your genes and, more often than not, that's a good thing. It's part of evolution's survival strategy.

Through a fascinating lifelong process of *epigenetic modulation*, some of your genes can be "turned on and off" according to your body's needs in response to changes in perceived environmental stressors. These changes in gene function do not change the DNA sequence, just the way it is expressed. Epigenetic changes occur in response to the presence or absence of nutrients, drugs, toxins, interpersonal stresses, and other factors.

Changes to the epigenome turn rigid genetic code into to an adaptive, environmentally sensitive instruction manual providing, in the best-case scenario, the body's protein-making machinery with the right directions at the right moment, while making sure all other instructions are suppressed. The "suppression" of the DNA code is every bit as important as the "expression" part, as every single cell in your body (except gametes and normal mature red blood cells) contains the genetic instructions to make everything. For example, a cell sitting at the tip of your nose contains a full set of DNA instructions for building muscle and creating eyeballs, while a brain cell has DNA instructions for filtering urine. Naturally, you do not want the nose cells to build an eyeball, and you certainly do not want brain cells processing urine. That's why suppressing what's not necessary or desirable is as crucial as expressing what is necessary.

You can think of epigenetics as a set of meta instructions modifying and revising the DNA manual throughout your life. Like DNA, the "meta" epigenetic manual is also inherited from your parents. Stressors during your lifetime and that of you parents and grandparents can change or add to this manual by helping you adapt to the ecosystem around you. The changes you accumulate can, in turn, be passed on to your children and grandchildren, which is one way living things evolve as a group and increase their chances of survival.

Three Kinds of Epigenetic Modulations

There are actually three kinds of epigenetic modulations: DNA methylation, histone modification, and microRNA regulation. The focus in this book will be on DNA methylation and how methyl donation is facilitated by vitamers.

Epigenetic Modulation

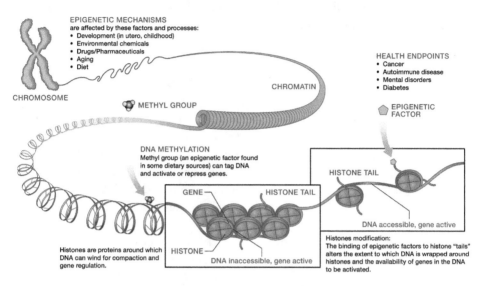

EPIGENETIC MECHANISMS
are affected by these factors and processes:
• Development (in utero, childhood)
• Environmental chemicals
• Drugs/Pharmaceuticals
• Aging
• Diet

CHROMOSOME

METHYL GROUP

CHROMATIN

HEALTH ENDPOINTS
• Cancer
• Autoimmune disease
• Mental disorders
• Diabetes

EPIGENETIC FACTOR

DNA METHYLATION
Methyl group (an epigenetic factor found in some dietary sources) can tag DNA and activate or repress genes.

HISTONE TAIL

GENE

HISTONE TAIL

DNA accessible, gene active

Histones are proteins around which DNA can wind for compaction and gene regulation.

HISTONE

DNA inaccessible, gene active

Histones modification:
The binding of epigenetic factors to histone "tails" alters the extent to which DNA is wrapped around histones and the availability of genes in the DNA to be activated.

How DNA Builds Proteins

The nuclei in the cells of your body contain some 25,000 to 35,000 genes, found inside threadlike strands called chromosomes. Each chromosome contains several thousand genes. These control cellular replication, providing the "blueprint" from which all proteins are made. The genes are made up of a structure called DNA. The recognizable double-helix shape of DNA strands looks like a long spiral staircase when uncoiled, with numerous connecting rods or steps evenly spaced between its two "banisters." What differentiates one piece of DNA from another is the order, number, and combination of four nucleotides serving as the connecting rods: adenine, thymine, cytosine, and guanine (A, T, C, and G, for short).

Any time a protein is needed, the DNA must unravel itself—at least, the section of DNA containing the gene for that protein—so it can be "read." Think of DNA as a thick instruction manual that must be opened to the proper page to get the correct instructions. Once the filaments are unraveled enough so the appropriate gene is readable, the genetic information is transcribed by an enzyme that makes another molecule, mRNA (messenger ribonucleic acid). The mRNA carries instructions out of the nucleus to macromolecular structures in the cytoplasm fluid of the cell called ribosomes. This is where proteins are made once the mRNA enters the ribosomes. Another enzyme translates the message, spelling out the exact length and order of the amino acids needed to build a specific protein. (All proteins are made out of combinations of various amino acids.)

Building a Human Being

The "building" of a fetus can be compared to the construction of a skyscraper. Both a fetus and a skyscraper have blueprints: one lies in the DNA, the other in the architect's drawings. When building a skyscraper, the blueprint is read by the builder, who issues instructions to the construction workers. In the fetus, it is RNA enzymes that "read" the genetic code of the DNA and carry this information to the ribosomes, the protein-manufacturing centers inside the cells.

For the skyscraper, some items in the architect's plans, such as drywall and electrical sockets, are used virtually everywhere, while others, like roof-tiles, are used only on the top. Likewise, in the fetus, some proteins in the body are used in virtually every cell, like the MTHFR enzyme, while others, like those used for color vision in the retina, are created only for a select set of cells. In both cases, the construction must be completed in a particular order. In a skyscraper, you can't put on the roof before you install the walls—and in the developing fetus, you can't create fingernails until there are fingers!

Epigenetics: Turning the Genes On and Off

DNA continually coils and uncoils itself, revealing one gene or several after another as necessary. What prompts the DNA to uncoil specific areas on demand? Thinking of it another way, what turns genes "on" so they can be read and "off" so they can't at just the right time? The process of turning genes on and off is called *gene expression*, and the mechanism by which that happens is called epigenetic methylation. Epi- means "on top of or in addition to"—epigenetic modifications are in addition to the genetic expression. The addition of a methyl group (a unit of one carbon atom plus three hydrogen atoms) attaching to the cytosine of the DNA is methylation. When a gene is expressed, its information is read and used to make proteins. When it is unexpressed, these proteins cannot be made, and the gene is said to be suppressed.

Many genes are always turned on because the body constantly needs to make the proteins they code for, such as red blood cell proteins. Others are almost always turned off, such as the genes that trigger breast cancer. About 30 percent of the genes in your body can be turned on or off as necessary. Some may be turned on only at a certain time during the day—for instance, the genes that program for sleep-inducing melatonin that is produced in higher amounts after the sun sets. Other genes are turned up or down at different times during the life cycle, such as those responsible for the production of estrogen or testosterone.

A great way to think of this epigenetic process is as a graduated on-and-off command system, like a volume knob on a radio. Epigenetics "tells" certain genes how much to be turned on (expressed) and how much to turn down (suppressed)—that is, when to reveal the instructions for making a protein and when to hide those instructions. So, epigenetics controls genetics. But what controls epigenetics?

Methylation Drives Epigenetics

The regulation of gene expression by the addition of a methyl group (methylation) to DNA is called *methylomics*. There are several cellular mechanisms regulating epigenetic expression this way, two of which are epigenetic methylation and histone modification. Epigenetic methylation works in response to our interaction with the environment and the resulting stressors, including availability (or lack) of nutrients, contact with pathogens, interpersonal stress, and exposure to noise, air pollution, and climate change. Put another way, what happens to us changes who we are.

A complex process, epigenetic methylation occurs when methyl groups attach to specific points on a gene. Once in place, these methyl groups prevent the DNA from being unraveled and read by the RNA-making enzyme, similar to a lock on a diary keeping the pages bound shut, unable to be read. As a result, no DNA can be interpreted, no messenger RNA can be made, and no protein can be produced. The gene is unread; it is suppressed—the gene cannot do what it is programmed to do.

Methyl groups don't actually block an individual gene; instead, they attract other methyl molecules because they "like" each other more than they "like" the water molecules around them (i.e., they are hydrophobic). This causes the DNA strands to pull together like magnets, sealing them shut if there are enough methyl groups donated by enough B vitamers.

DNA: The "Barcode" of Body Parts

To understand how DNA, RNA, and methylation function, think about the check-out process at a modern coffee shop. The bar code you have on your phone for your specialty coffee drink can be viewed as the "set in stone" DNA, unless there has been a misprint (mutation). The scanner at the register reads the barcode just like the RNA enzyme reads the DNA. The scanner then sends an electrical signal messenger RNA (mRNA) to the barista (ribosomes) in the back. She reads your request, brings together the ingredients, and creates one of a limited number of coffee options (proteins) she then delivers to you. Methylation is like a piece of tape covering the bar code: no information can be read or printed, and no mocha lattes (proteins) will be made.

In general, increased methylation turns certain genes off, while a reduction of methylation allows them to be turned on. This makes methylation a natural and necessary process playing an important role in normal embryonic development, gene silencing, keeping certain cancers at bay, repairing DNA errors, and aiding in long-term memory storage, among many other things. There are methyl groups scattered all over your DNA, with epigenetic methylation acting on about one-third of your body's protein-producing genes, or about 7,000 in all. A methyl group will only attach itself to a specific place on the DNA molecule, where cytosine and guanine occur as a pair. If a gene happens to have a lot of these cytosine-guanine pairs, it is more likely to be controlled by the methylation process.

B12 and folate are essential for proper methylation because the two vitamers are crucial for converting homocysteine into SAMe, a major methyl donor to DNA. If B12 and folate are deficient in the diet or poorly absorbed, the methylation process will suffer—and so will you.

You Are What Your Grandparents Ate

Genetic expression is often described as being completely turned on or off, but it would be more accurate to describe it as "turned up" or "turned down" like the flame on a gas stove. Where the "knob" is set depends on current or past stresses, whether they are environmental, psychological, health-oriented, or financial, just to name several. These epigenetic influences can then become embedded in the "cellular memory" and last throughout the life of the individual, and maybe on through subsequent generations.

By reviewing research started after World War II, we can see how the multigenerational impact of B-vitamer deprivation started. During the brutal winter of 1944–45, the German army drastically cut back on food deliveries to the occupied western Netherlands, setting off a six-month period of severe starvation for the Dutch people living in the area. This famine, known as *Hongerwinter* ("hunger winter"), affected around 4.5 million people. During the worst of it, many were living on as little as 500 calories a day. Malnutrition was rampant, and some 22,000 people died of starvation.

Horrific as the famine was, it did provide a fascinating natural study of the effects of maternal starvation on children exposed to famine in utero during the first ten weeks following conception. Compared to their unexposed same-sex siblings, the exposed children, who are now close to seventy-five years old, have had a greater rate of death due to the increased risk of diabetes, obesity, and schizophrenia.[25]

Even more startling is the fact these increased risks were inherited by their children, the grandchildren of the starved pregnant women. By way of comparison, those who were in utero just *before* or *after* the starvation had a normal mortality rate, which means that there was something about that particular ten-week period in utero that set up generations for unhealthy aging and premature death.

We now know the increased risk of disease among the in-the-womb *Hongerwinter* children and their offspring was caused by the expression during early gestation of a specific gene called insulin-like growth factor-2 (IGF2). While maternal starvation did not cause changes to the DNA coding for the IGF2 gene itself, the lack of B12 and folate did change the *epigenetic* way that gene was expressed.

These epigenetic changes were survival-positive at the time, for they made the unborn children and the newborn children better able to hold on to every single calorie provided by their starving mothers. When the food supply was reestablished, the children continued to latch on to every single carbohydrate calorie possible. This ratcheted up their risk of developing obesity and obesity-related diseases such as diabetes, even seven decades later. And these epigenetic changes were also programmed into the tiny egg cells growing within the female fetuses' ovaries during that terrible winter, which is how the changes were passed on into the next generation.[26]

---

[25] Columbia University's Mailman School of Public Health, "Prenatal Exposure to Famine May Lead to Persistent Epigenetic Changes," *Science Daily*, November 3, 2008.

[26] The study did not examine whether the epigenetic changes were passed on through males.

Epigenetics plays out in complex ways, many we have yet to discover. Yet it is clear that what we do and what happens to us in our lifetime influences the way our genes are expressed, and these changes can be passed on to future generations. While our well-known immediate response to stressors is to fight, flee, or freeze, epigenetic changes in gene expression is our long-term response, one that says, "Get ready for the next time you or your children experience this threat!"

Methylation You Can See–the Agouti Gene Mice

Remember the agouti gene mice I talked about in chapter one? Their odd yellow fur is evidence of reduced epigenetic methylation, because the agouti gene also controls coloring. Agouti mice are normally a mousy brown color. When a pregnant agouti mouse is deliberately deprived of folate in her diet, less methylation will occur within her cells. Decreased methylation translates to decreased suppression (and increased expression) of the agouti gene, and as a consequence, the mice grow yellow fur.

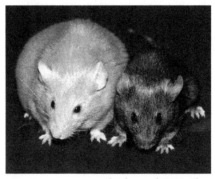

Agouti gene mice with identical DNA. The one on the left was born of a mother with low levels of prenatal folate, resulting in low levels of methylation and low agouti gene suppression. (Image by R. Jirtle/ D. Dolinoy 2007 and used in compliance with creative commons attribution 3.0 unported license.)

Agouti mice genetics also allow for less suppression of a gene that increases the breakdown of fats. This means that fat builds up, and the yellow-furred mice develop obesity. These little yellow fur-balls look nothing like their slim, dark-furred siblings, born when their mother was fed a nutritious mouse diet. The yellow-furred mice show more susceptibility to diabetes, cancer, and several other diseases than their siblings—and all because their mothers lacked folate in their prenatal diets! For these mice, less folate vitamer meant less methylation, leading to increased expression of previously repressed genes. In equation form, it looks like this:

$$\downarrow \text{Folate} \rightarrow \downarrow \text{Methylation} \rightarrow \downarrow \text{Agouti Gene Suppression}$$
$$(\uparrow \text{expression}) \rightarrow \uparrow \text{Obesity, Diabetes, Cancer, Death}$$

It's long been suspected that epigenetic methylation, or a lack thereof, is not simply nutrition related. Certain environmental factors play a role as well. Testing this theory, Dr. Randy Jirtle from the University of Wisconsin looked beyond folate deprivation to the effects of bisphenol-A (BPA) on agouti gene expression. BPA, a common environmental pollutant found in baby bottles and other plastic containers,[27] is known to specifically disrupt genes and hormones. When Dr. Jirtle fed healthy pregnant agouti mice a normal mouse diet plus BPA, a startling 31 percent of the offspring were born with yellow fur, became obese, and had higher rates of diabetes and cancer during their lifetimes. This indicates that BPA exposure suppressed methylation of the agouti gene. However, when mice with a suppressed agouti gene (meaning they were yellow and obese) became pregnant and were fed diets high in folate, their offspring were well methylated and had brown fur and healthy, normal lifespans.

The implication is that consuming a methyl-rich diet prevented the negative epigenetic changes suffered by the mother from being expressed in the offspring. It also means that the diet and supplements your mother ingested during pregnancy may still affect you (for better or for worse) to this day!

The Challenge of Having Two X Chromosomes

Methylation is essential, not only for the sequencing of cell development and gene expression, but also for the timing of hormonal production, especially at the onset of puberty. Up until that point, the genes allowing sex hormone production have been turned way down and kept fairly quiet by a phenomenon called *gene silencing*. When precise signaling from inside the cell and from other cells is coordinated, the methylation block is lifted, the genes are allowed to fully express themselves, estrogen and testosterone manufacturing is thrown into high gear, and *voila!* puberty begins.

One important example of gene silencing pertains to females only because

---

[27] Dolinoy D.C., Huang D., Jirtle R.L., Maternal Nutrient Supplementation Counteracts Bisphenol A-Induced DNA Hypomethylation in Early Development, *Proc Natl Acad Sci U.S.A.* 2007; 104(32):13056–61.

they have two X chromosomes, instead of the single X males have. Half of female "double X" genes must be inactivated, or the female body will make twice the necessary amount of proteins, both "good" and "bad." Thus, the appropriate DNA segment on one of the X-chromosomes must be methylated to prevent that gene from "double-expressing" itself. A substandard diet, inadequate supplements, and/or poor health can lead to hypomethylation (a lack of available methyl groups), resulting in an increased production of the proteins expressed by the redundant X. Since many genes controlling the immune response are located on the X chromosome, females with hypomethylation who express both Xs can suffer from overactive immune responses, resulting in higher rates of autoimmune illnesses such as rheumatoid arthritis, lupus, celiac disease, and many others.[28] Because males don't have the challenge of double expression of genes, they have much lower overall rates of autoimmune illness, but they are more susceptible to infections because they have a more sluggish inflammatory response with just one X.

Have It Your (Epigenetic) Way

A new approach to medical therapeutics is just getting started: nutritional epigenetics, or the modification of genetic expression through the use of dietary adjustments, vitamer supplementation, environmental changes, and other means of fine-tuning one's nutrient status. (More about this in later chapters.) Here is an example of how dietary changes can alter epigenetic legacy.

Adipose tissue (fat cells) uses more than its share of folate, so those who have an excess number of cells often have less folate available for use in methylation. This makes individuals more susceptible to health issues associated with hypomethylation, such as heart disease, dementia, cancer, diabetes, and kidney disease. As mentioned above, the tendency toward all of these diseases can not only be developed by the mother, but also can be passed on to her unborn children. Interestingly, it's been found that when women undergo gastric bypass surgeries and lose weight before becoming pregnant, the hypomethylation health risks to their offspring are diminished. Thus, in this instance and others, it is actually possible to rewrite a bad epigenetic legacy that might have been in place for generations!

The positive effects of prenatal B12 and folate supplementation on methylation and, therefore, the health of the offspring, might look like this in equation form:

---

[28] Fairweather, D., "Sex Differences in Autoimmune Disease from a Pathological Perspective," *American Journal of Pathology*, September 2008, 173(3):600–9.

↑Pre-natal B12/F→↑Methylation→↑Suppression of Bad
Genes→↓Obesity, ↓Diabetes, ↓Cancer

A summation of the importance of the study of hypomethylation can best be distilled down to the following concise quote by Drs. Pogribny, et al. where they state:

> The pathogenesis of any given human disease is a complex multifactorial process characterized by many biologically significant and interdependent alterations. One of these changes, specific to a wide range of human pathologies, is DNA hypomethylation. It is clear that disease by itself can induce hypomethylation of DNA; however, a decrease in DNA methylation can also have an impact on the predisposition to pathological states and disease development. This review presents evidence suggesting the involvement of DNA hypomethylation in the pathogenesis of several major human pathologies, including cancer, atherosclerosis, Alzheimer's disease, and psychiatric disorders.[29]

An Epigenetic Aging Clock?

Epigenetic methylation is absolutely critical to the length and quality of our lives, yet predictable decreases in the degree of methylation of DNA occur with aging. These decreases have also been linked to disease. Colorectal cancer was the first epigenetic disease identified in 1983, when researchers found that the affected tissues had decreased DNA methylation, leading to atypical protein formation. Since that time, studies have linked faulty DNA methylation to many other diseases and conditions, including neurological and cardiovascular disorders, childhood leukemia, allergies, asthma, fetal alcohol syndrome, childhood obesity, type 2 diabetes, reproductive problems, and aging.[30]

Recently, Dr. Steven Horvath of UCLA developed an "age predictor" that measures DNA methylation at 353 specific gene sites known to have age-associated increases or decreases in methyl groups. Dr. Horvath then computed a "biological age" at each site, which is sometimes referred to as "Horvath's

---

[29] Pogribny, I., et al, DNA Hypomethylation in the Origin and Pathogenesis of Human Diseases, *Cellular and Molecular Life Sciences,* July 2009, Vol. 66, Issue 14.
[30] Rodenhiser D, Mann M., "Epigenetics and Human Disease: Translating Basic Biology into Clinical Applications," *CMAJ,* 2006;174:341–348. Also see http://pedsinreview.aappublications.org/content/36/1/14].

Clock." He discovered that methylation occurs more quickly between birth and adulthood, then slows to a constant rate. However, when problems such as breast cancer develop, the cells begin aging faster, and their "methylation age" can exceed the age of normal breast cells by as much as thirty-six years! This means that different parts of your body might be aging at different rates.[31] This leads to an obvious question: If the availability of methyl groups affects epigenetics, what kind of intracellular signaling system controls when and where the methyl groups are placed? The researcher who figures this out should get a Nobel Prize.

What's the Next Step Beyond Epigenetic Methylation?

In summary, the availability of sufficient numbers of methyl groups is key to epigenetic methylation, a process that ensures the timely expression or suppression of certain genes. SAMe is a major donor of methyl groups, and B12 and folate are crucial to its production. Too little B12 or folate may result in too little SAMe, which in turn will suppress epigenetic methylation. Insufficient methylation can allow "bad" genes, previously kept silent, to express themselves, leading to a host of diseases, including neurological and cardiovascular disorders, allergies, asthma, childhood obesity, type 2 diabetes, and unhealthy aging.

What is the one thing all of these terrible diseases have in common, besides hypomethylation? An all-too-prevalent condition everyone should be wary of, which is even more dangerous when we are lacking B12 and folate: chronic inflammation.

---

[31] Horvath, S., "DNA Methylation Age of Human Tissues and Cell Types," *Genome Biology*, 2013;14:3156.

SIX

STRESSED OUT AND STRESSED IN

↑Stressors→↑Stress →↓Homeostasis→
↑Inflammation →Unhealthy Aging/Death

Fresh out of medical school, I embarked on my first rotation as part of a pediatric internship in a big-city hospital emergency room. Called upon to examine a toddler one night, I began by reading the chart, which documented that this active little boy had developed a high fever due to an infected wound where a large splinter of wood had punctured deep into his thigh muscles. The toddler's parents had removed the splinter, but they weren't sure they got it all. Over the course of the next several days, the area became red, warm, swollen, and painful when touched—classic signs of inflammation and infection. Soon after, his parents noticed a small boil had formed where they had pulled out the splinter. After his fever spiked and he refused liquids, his mother brought him to the emergency room.

Upon entering the examining room, I was alarmed by the demeanor of the toddler. He laid placidly on the exam table, absolutely silent, watching me with big, sad eyes. When a sick young child in a doctor's office gives up on crying, you know something is terribly wrong.

Although I didn't yet realize it, the little boy was dying—dying of stress. Not the kind of stress you experience in traffic or when chewed out by your boss, but stress in its broadest and most correct definition: the body's response to any stressor knocking it out of equilibrium, out of homeostasis. And this young child's stress was devastating. After heroic efforts—medical and surgical—he died of an overwhelming infection prompting his liver, kidneys, and nervous system to shut down, one by one. The splinter was the stressor, and his body's response was the stress. (I will describe the wide variety of stressors we are exposed to in later chapters.)

Every disease and *every* physical or emotional assault upon the body upsets its equilibrium and triggers a stress response. This stress causes the natural inflammatory process to ramp up to levels potentially causing significant problems. To regain equilibrium, the body must spend a lot of biochemical energy. In tens of millions of us, the disruption to our internal equilibrium with the resulting inflammation is slowly but surely damaging our health. The solution doesn't lie in taking another medicine or undergoing surgery. The solution is to reduce the long-term over-response to stressors as much as possible. I am suggesting the vitamers of B12 and folate are vital in the fight to return to a healthy homeostasis.

Confusing Nomenclature

The word *stress* is often used to identify something that assails or upsets us, as well as the resulting effect(s) on the body and the way we feel about it. Thus, stress may describe being caught in traffic and the resulting increase in blood pressure and the urge to honk nastily at every car in sight. Indeed, stress has become a multipurpose, difficult-to-define word whose meaning is often evident only from the context. (Just trying to define the word is stressful!)

For the purposes of our discussion, *stress* is the situation arising when the body's equilibrium has experienced a "stressor," and a *stressor* is anything causing a stress response. Part of the stress response is the body's effort to return to a homeostatic state. A stressor can be just about anything—a germ, a physical injury, a perceived threat, another person, a situation, a feeling, a severe change in temperature, an excess or lack of food, or the loss of a loved one. Stress is the body's attempt to right itself.

I call *stressing out* what can be observed by others and felt by you. I call *stressing in* the damage done to your physiology over the long term. This damage is often not felt or observed until irreparable harm has occurred.

The Universal Illness

Although innumerable studies have shown the dangers, even deadliness, of excessive stress, it's difficult to understand how such a wide variety of medical problems are caused by it. After all, stress-related conditions such as heart disease, depression, and cancer are all very different, with different origins and methods of progression. How can stress cause the clogged arteries seen in heart disease, plus the changes in brain wave patterns characteristic of depression, plus the wildly multiplying cells known as cancer? To answer this question, we need to push beyond the specifics of a single disease to consider the challenge stressors pose to the body's equilibrium. No matter what the stressor, it triggers increased production of certain stress hormones and white blood cells with the suppression of others. Stressors interrupt normal brain-wave patterns and alter the behavior of the immune system. In short, stressors knock the body out of balance. This upset in homeostasis, and the body's attempt to reestablish it, is what harms us. Clearly, there's a lot more to stress than a temporary rise in blood pressure or the feeling of being so overwhelmed you have to lie down.

Unfortunately, knowledge about stress-stressor responses remains limited. For example, medical students have long been taught that stress triggers heart disease by ratcheting up blood pressure and cholesterol levels, damaging the interior walls of the arteries supplying blood to the heart muscle. Eventually this damage results in a clot large enough to block the flow of blood through the capillary vessels of the heart, triggering a heart attack. Your doctor first does as he should and recommends eating better, exercising more, and losing weight. He knows from your chart that he has given you these suggestions many times over the years, and you have chosen not to follow them. As a consequence, the next step you have unintentionally chosen is medication or surgery and the side-effects associated with these.

Let's compare this to the shaking a house receives during an earthquake. Imagine that you live in Oklahoma and nearby fracking (stressor) for oil is causing earthquakes (heart attack, strokes). Depending on how severe the shaking is, the lights flicker a little, pictures fall, dishes tumble out of the cabinets, walls lean out of plumb, the foundation cracks, or perhaps the entire house collapses.

These can be serious problems, but once the quake has subsided, it would be ridiculous for the contractor to declare that the house is suffering from "sclerosis of the walls" because the walls crumbled—or diagnose it with a severe case of "MFCS (Multiple Foundation Crack Syndrome)" because the foundation cracked. The real problem was obviously the stressor—fracking—caused combined damage (stress) in areas of specific weaknesses in the construction of the house. The solution, then, is to restore the house's equilibrium by repairing its foundation, shoring up its walls, and so on, so it can withstand the next earthquake. Yet this still won't treat the fracking, which is the underlying cause of the cracked walls and foundation—an analogy here for chronic inflammation.

Unfortunately, people with stress-related diseases such as heart disease tend to focus solely on the obvious results of the disequilibrium, such as elevated cholesterol or blood pressure. They ignore the underlying foundation entirely. They are missing the real issue—the fact that the body is out of homeostasis—which eventually shows up as the universal illness: inflammation.

Holding Things Dynamically Constant

The concept of the body being maintained in a dynamic balance was introduced back in 1876 when the renowned physiologist Dr. Claude Bernard proposed the concept of *milieu interieur*, or "internal milieu." According to Dr. Bernard, health depends on maintaining a fairly fixed internal environment; body temperature, blood oxygen, blood glucose, and other physiologic measures must remain within narrow ranges.

Think of a tire on your car. Its internal milieu consists of its air pressure, which must remain within a certain range. If the pressure falls too low, the tire goes flat; while if it climbs too high, the tire bursts. In addition, the tire's rubber must maintain a certain integrity and flexibility. A thin tire wall will be easily punctured. A too-thick and rigid wall will make for a hard ride. The tire works best when proper amounts of air pressure, rubber integrity, and rubber flexibility are maintained.

The same concept can be applied to the human body—although, unlike the tire, your body has defenses against challenges to its internal milieu. For example, when blood sugar falls too low, your body triggers the release of stored energy, bringing blood sugar levels back into appropriate range. The ability to maintain an internal milieu, a homeostasis, is what separates the non-living from the living. All living things have this ability, from the simplest single-cell bacteria all the way up to the amazingly complex human being.

The word *homeostasis* was coined in 1932 by Dr. Walter Cannon to describe the complex positive and negative feedback system the body uses to defend its internal environment. Derived from Greek, *homeostasis* means "similar to standing still." This literal translation highlights a key concept: Homeostasis doesn't mean remaining absolutely still, unchanging and unmoving. Instead, it suggests that while any particular body measurement—such as the blood oxygen level—might look static when you check it, there are many counterbalancing dynamic forces keeping measurements at a specific set point, or within a desired range.

Consider a helium balloon on a string. The weight differential of helium inside the balloon and the air outside is "telling" the balloon to rise, but the string you are holding in your hand is "telling" it not to. The upward force of the helium and the downward force of your hand on the string are equally balanced, so the balloon remains where it is, suspended in the air by the counterbalancing forces. While at any given moment the balloon might rise or fall a tiny bit, it remains more or less in place unless some stressor changes the equilibrium.

Homeostasis, then, is the maintenance of a balanced state within a complex, interdependent system, with the balance secured by numerous positive and negative feedback loops.

Homeostasis Is a Balancing Act

The figure below shows just one homeostatic balance point or, more accurately, a single positive/negative feedback loop: the fasting blood glucose (sugar) level. Ideally, the fasting level should be about 90 mg/dl. Blood glucose doesn't simply find this level and remain there. At any given time, forces exert upward pressure, such as release of carbohydrates from recently eaten food, while increasing insulin production that facilitates glucose movement into the cell exerts a downward pressure on levels. In this example, the "up" and "down" forces balance out, holding blood glucose levels at about 90 mg/dl, resulting in a healthy homeostasis.

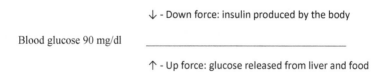

↓ - Down force: insulin produced by the body

Blood glucose 90 mg/dl _____

↑ - Up force: glucose released from liver and food

Now imagine additional "up forces" in blood glucose levels such as weight gain, decreased exercise, psychological stress, and inflammation, while the "down force" of insulin production stays the same. These "up forces" overwhelm the single "down force," and blood glucose levels rise.

↓ Down force: insulin production

New glucose level: 120 mg/dl _____

↑ - Up force: food, weight gain, decreased exercise,

psychological stress, inflammation

If the new "up forces" remain and no new "down forces" are added, the blood glucose levels will remain permanently elevated, becoming the new homeostasis—the new normal. A new "normal" is not necessarily a healthy new normal and in this case is prediabetic.

Of course, this higher glucose homeostasis is not an isolated measurement. Everything in your body—from bacteria in the gut to the complex motor cortex in the brain—is interconnected. Whatever happens in one part of your body reverberates throughout the whole, no matter how insignificant it might seem. For example, this new, higher blood glucose level increases inflammation throughout your body. Increased inflammation, then, becomes an "up factor" or a "down factor" in numerous other homeostatic points such as blood pressure, cholesterol production, or wound healing.

This brings us to a key point: Homeostasis is not a single, specific item identified and measured. Instead, there are thousands and thousands of homeostatic balance points besides glucose levels within the body. Some of these include oxygen balance, body temperature maintenance, cancer-cell suppression, and B12/F absorption. All are interrelated and interdependent. The aberrant rise or fall of a single point puts pressure on others, sometimes many others, possibly causing a cascade of negative events. The reverse is also true. Restoring a single homeostatic balance point to its healthy level can relieve pressure on numerous other points, leading to better health. A recent study[32] by researcher Ana Arigony and her colleagues claims that certain nutrients, including B12 and folate, are critical to all DNA pathways and thus homeostasis. They state: "Without the proper nutrients, genomic instability compromises homeostasis, leading to chronic diseases and certain types of cancer."

Stressing the Points

Stressors can be defined as anything having the potential to knock the body

---

[32] Arigony, A.L.V., de Oliveira, J.M., Machado, M., et al, "The Influence of Micronutrients in Cell Culture: A Reflection on Viability and Genomic Stability," *BioMed Research International*, 2013; Article ID 597282.

out of homeostasis. Whether it's in the form of a poor diet increasing blood glucose/fat levels, a miserable interpersonal relationship sending blood pressure soaring, a bacterial invasion, or a broken bone, if it disturbs the body's equilibrium, it is a stressor.

The greater the stressor, the greater the stress response, the harder the body must work to regain homeostasis, and the greater the odds one or more of an individual's less-secure homeostatic balance points will be affected. Perhaps the weak link is cholesterol control, or blood pressure, or the ability to sleep through the night. Perhaps it's a genetic tendency toward allergies or obesity. Whatever the propensity may be, stressors usually "find" the weak points with the stress response of inflammation. This is the reason stress can trigger so many different kinds of disease symptoms and life problems.

Perhaps the most classic form of inflammation, and the easiest to visualize, is the body's response to a pathogenic invasion. When a bacterium enters the body, it is rapidly detected by the immune system, which sends out the physiological version of a SEAL quick-response team, followed by backup ground troops. Immune system cells, constantly "on patrol," are the first to detect the invader and send out chemical messages alerting the rest of the immune system. Other immune system cells quickly join the fray and send messages describing the invader to a specific part of the immune system. This area fashions a certain kind of white cells called B-cells, specifically designed to destroy a particular pathogen—physiologic "smart bombs," if you will.

In addition to the fighting immune cells and the "smart bombs," the immune system sends "controller cells" to the area to help direct the fight by calling for more immune soldiers when necessary and instructing those engaged in battle to back off at the appropriate time. Once the invader has been destroyed, the controller cells direct the cleanup effort, and soon everything is back to a normal balance. Thanks to the inflammatory process, homeostasis has been restored.

But things are not always ideal. Sometimes the invader overwhelms the body's attempt to defend itself, as happened with my young patient with the thigh wound. Sometimes the body's defense system itself becomes the problem. Allergies, which result from the body's misguided attempt to maintain homeostasis, are an example of this.

One Sunday afternoon, while working in the pediatric ER, I evaluated a fourteen-year old girl who had been rushed in from a church picnic. She was suffering from rapidly progressing respiratory distress because exposure to peanuts (the stressor) had caused an allergic reaction (the stress response).

While she had had mild reactions in the past, this current response was much worse. When I entered the room, she was sitting straight up with a tight grip on the edge of the stretcher, using her voluntary breathing muscles to take in air and force it back out. Even with oxygen flowing through a tube into her nose, she was working very hard to breathe and rapidly becoming exhausted, with her lips turning blue.

The unfortunate girl was suffering from a peanut allergy. As soon as the peanut protein entered her body, her immune system hit the panic button, turning its full wrath on what it interpreted as the "invader." As part of her body's defense procedure, her immune response had released powerful pro-inflammatory hormones that, unfortunately, caused her trachea to swell. Its opening became more and more restricted, leaving less room for the flow of air.

It was not little pieces of peanut blocking her windpipe causing the problem but her body's over-response to the proteins in the peanuts. The girl's system was knocked way out of homeostasis by a flood of pro-inflammatory, trachea-closing hormones. By the time I saw her, her body was trying to produce enough anti-inflammatory hormones, such as cortisol, to help the trachea disengorge and reopen. She was losing the fight, and her swollen windpipe was strangling her, just as surely as if someone's hands were around her throat. Fortunately, an injection of epinephrine reversed the inflammatory response in minutes. Her tracheal tissues shrank to normal size, and she was soon breathing easily.

Think You've Had a Bad Day?

In 2014, Australian Rod Sommerville was bitten by one of the deadliest snakes in the world—an eastern brown snake. He called for an ambulance, then grabbed a cold beer and sat down to drink while waiting for either help or death, whichever came first. Help arrived, and he was given an anti-venom serum just in time to stop the fatal nerve toxin. The only problem was that he developed a life-threatening allergic reaction to the anti-venom serum, and he had to be re-saved.

Terrible as they can be, allergic reactions are usually treatable if caught in time. More dangerous is the often-subtle damage arising when the body tries to maintain homeostasis and the process goes awry. Coronary artery disease is a good example of this. In many cases the problem begins with cytokines, chemical messengers present in all immune responses. Cytokines are excreted by many kinds of cells throughout the body and brain. When an invading virus, for example, enters the bloodstream, cells lining interior blood vessel walls become inflamed and release cytokines. The inflamed cells do not swell, as you might expect, but instead shrink in size. Rather than forming a tightly packed wall, they become a "leaky" wall with lots of "spaces" through which extracellular fluids flow. The fluid sloshing between the cell walls brings with it more cytokines, along with additional immune cells. These white blood cells include the giant macrophages, which roam around looking for diseased and dying cells to engulf and digest.

Cell shrinkage and resulting "leaky" walls are a necessary part of the inflammatory process, but the body thinks something is wrong with the cells, so it sends in even more cytokines and macrophages, plus the hormone cortisol. The cortisol instructs the body to increase cholesterol production in the bloodstream to more efficiently make new cells and store energy (fat) for the long healing process ahead. When stress (inflammation) overwhelms cells lining the blood vessels in the heart, they become damaged or die. Cholesterol then plugs the gaps and atherosclerotic plaques form, causing the blood vessel walls to thicken and narrow, damaging interior vessel linings of the vessels even more, leading to reduced blood flow. Now you have the narrowed arteries associated with heart attacks, strokes, dementia, and accelerated aging. These diseases weren't caused simply by eating too many fatty foods, and they weren't caused by elevated blood pressure. They were caused by the inflammatory process initiated by the introduction of the stressors—in this case bad diet and high blood pressure.

This scenario doesn't account for all cases of heart attack, strokes, and dementia, but it does explain how millions of cases get started or are made worse. Unfortunately, the medical response is often too late in the treatment process.

All Stressors Challenge Homeostasis and Trigger Inflammation

It's not just physical injuries, germ invasions, or allergies triggering stress and inflammation; emotional distress can do the same. To understand this let's go back to 1932, when Dr. Walter Cannon ran into a problem while studying the digestive process of pigeons. Every time he entered his lab, the door creaked, startling the birds. Their heart rates soared, their digestion stopped, and the frustrated doctor had to start his experiment all over again and again.

Dr. Cannon became intrigued by the connection between emotional distress—the startle response he triggered by the opening door—and the cessation of digestion. Through a classic, still-studied experiment, he discovered that when with the startle response was activated, nerves running from the brain to the heart trigger an increase in heart rate. Even when those nerves were cut, the heart rate still increased, leading him to believe the heart was stimulated by something else, perhaps something in the blood. Through a process of elimination, Dr. Cannon discovered that if he removed the adrenal glands from an animal whose "startle response" nerves had been cut, their heart rates did not soar when he alarmed them. Therefore, he deduced, the adrenal glands must be the source of a chemical messenger stimulating the heart, and he named the substance after the gland producing it: *adrenalin.*

This discovery led to our current understanding of how the body responds to anything it perceives as dangerous—from the sudden appearance of a snarling dog to riding on a roller coaster; from awaiting the results of an important test to suddenly seeing a flashing blue or red light in your rearview mirror. This "Warning, Warning!" thought is processed by the medulla, a primitive part of the brain responsible for basic functions such as breathing, heart rate, and blood pressure. The information is then transmitted to the higher-functioning cerebrum for conscious interpretation of the stressor, as well as to the hypothalamus for unconscious processing.

Dr. Cannon found that the almond-sized hypothalamus, nestled in the middle of the brain, transmits signals to the rest of the body in two ways. The first is through direct nerve stimulation of various organs via the sympathetic nervous system (SNS). The SNS is a collection of nerves, the function of which is to get the body ready to either fight or run for its life. The SNS is responsible for hyperarousal symptoms, including increases in the heart and respiration rates, blood pressure, blood sugar, serum fat, bladder urgency, and blood clotting, as well as decreased digestion and reduced sex drive.

The second mechanism is via hormonal activation by the hypothalamus and the pituitary gland, the fundamental hormonal facilitators between the brain and body. The B_{12}/folate-rich pituitary sends out hormones that stimulate endocrine glands throughout the body, including the adrenals, ovaries, testes, thyroid, and bone marrow. (This pathway is called the Hypothalamus-Pituitary-Adrenal axis, or HPA axis.) Bear in mind that if the pituitary gland is not able to maintain its high concentration of B_{12}/F, the efficiency of the HPA axis is negatively affected, as is the inflammatory response required.

Upon receiving the appropriate signals via the HPA axis, the endocrine glands respond by releasing their own hormones, cytokines, macrophages, and cortisol into the bloodstream. In a very real sense, this is an inflammatory response complete with the release of clotting factors for plugging any possible blood vessel leaks (injuries).

Hypothalamic - Pituitary - Adrenal Axis

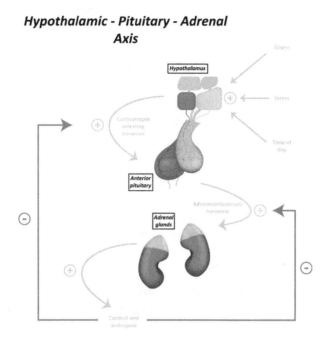

What an amazing concept: Your body's response to a nasty dog snarling at you is essentially an inflammatory response, even though nothing has touched you or breached your skin barrier. Indeed, the dog could turn out to be quite friendly and the danger completely illusory, but your brief burst of fear is still taken seriously by your body when it initiates the inflammatory sequence. This happens in case an injury should occur and healing becomes necessary.

In short, the human body was designed to respond to *every* challenge, whether it is physical, perceptual, or emotional, with an inflammatory response. That's great, because inflammation is a vital part of the body's defense and repair mechanisms. And that's also terrible, because too much inflammation is dangerous, often deadly.

Stewing in Inflammation Devastates Health

Our ancient ancestors faced plenty of stressors, but at least they could either engage in battle or run like heck, and once the danger had passed, their pituitary glands, hypothalamus, and other body parts could bring their body chemistry back into homeostasis. Today we're subject to endless physical assaults—from germs, air pollution, and man-made chemicals to emotional assaults in the form of crowding, unpleasant workplaces, traffic, and more. All of these can trigger a flood of powerful fight-or-flight substances—increasing heart rate, respiratory rate, blood pressure, and blood sugar and causing the release of fats and blood-clotting factors, all while suppressing digestion and sex drive. Yet more often than not, we are unable to either fight or flee and are stuck with a third choice: freeze. We are then locked in a state of hyperarousal with no way to "burn off" the chemical stew roiling inside. And the "freeze response" is killing us just as surely as fighting ever did.

The "freeze response" has a definite role in our modern world. When your boss yells at you, it's probably not a great idea to put up your dukes or turn and run away. It exacts a price. Getting stuck in a state of stress hyperarousal over the long term can manifest as irritability, anger, depression, poor sleep, decreased sex drive, intestinal symptoms, and fatigue. All of these are harmful to the body and, crucially, all interfere with the normal inflammation process. When a chronic low level of inflammation is maintained, a healthy response becomes less available when "real" stressors appear. Maladaptive attempts to lessen the irritability, depression, and anxiety of stress by taking it out on ourselves (self-medicating, overeating) or taking it out on others (aggression) can be much more harmful than the initial stressor.

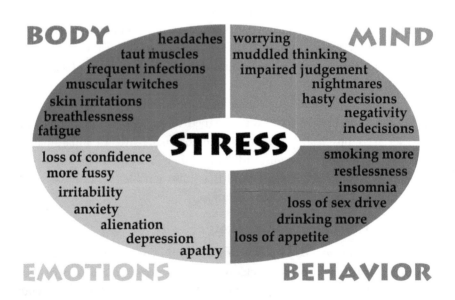

Accelerated Immunosenescence

Our ability to keep inflammation in the "homeostatic sweet spot" naturally declines with age. This reduction, called *immunosenescence*, is a normal part of aging, just as are loss of musculature, lower hormone levels, and dimmer vision. Unfortunately, living with chronic low-level inflammation, as so many of us do, speeds up the decline. Without enough B12 and folate, the acceleration into unhealthy aging is even greater.

In Sum: The Universal Illness Is "Stressor-Induced Inflammation"

The body's reaction to a stressor (whether physical or emotional) and the resulting upset to homeostasis *is* the inflammatory response. This includes the flooding of the body with powerful fight-or-flight substances that increase heart rate, respiratory rate, blood pressure, blood sugar, release of fats, and blood-clotting factors, among other things. This response is necessary to healing, but unfortunately, when it's out of control, it can damage or even kill us.

The solution is not to design a new surgery or pill but to reduce stressors by helping the body maintain homeostasis via tamping down any unnecessary or exaggerated inflammatory responses. Until we do all of these, we may as well slap a bandage on some very serious conditions. And I do mean serious: According to the Centers for Disease Control and Prevention, the ten leading causes of death for Americans are heart disease, cancer, chronic respiratory disease, accidents, strokes, Alzheimer's disease, diabetes, influenza and pneumonia, kidney disease, and suicide.[33] Signs of inflammation have been found as components of every one of these causes except death by accidents. (Even many of those accidents, however, have an emotional component.)

Focused on finding the single problem causing each disease—a specific germ, genetic error, injury, or malfunction—medical science has missed the hidden truth about stress for a long time. Inflammation is the foundation of most illness even when the onset is caused by other stressors (genetics, infection), and it could rightly be called the *universal illness*. Taming it should be an integral part of any treatment program.

---

[33] Centers for Disease Control and Prevention, Injury Prevention & Control: *Data & Statistics (WISQARS)*. "10 Leading Causes of Death by Age Group, United States—2014," Accessible at http://www.cdc.gov/injury/wisqars/pdf/leading causes of death by age group 2014-a.pdf. June 27, 2016.

SEVEN

INFLAMED

↑Abiotic Stressors→↑Biotic Stressors→
↑Psychological Stressors→↑Inflammation→Unhealthy Aging

As covered in the previous chapter, stress is a physiologic state arising when the body's equilibrium is upset. The stress state is followed by the body's efforts to restore baseline homeostasis. The stress state is initiated by a challenge, a stressor that may be one of three types—biotic, abiotic, or psychological. Although these three types of stressors are very different, they all trigger the stress response, increasing the inflammatory load and the risk of unhealthy aging.

Stressors in the Form of Biotic Challenges

A biotic stressor is any stressor that is living, comes alive once it enters the body, or was made by a living organism. Viruses, bacteria, parasites, and biotoxins sharing the environment with us can be biotic stressors. Some are commonplace, like the *Staphylococcus* bacteria always sitting on your skin, ready to dive into your body if you cut yourself. Some viruses are commonplace like influenza, and some are exotic, transmitted to us by animals, including Ebola and Corona from bats, Chikungunya from mosquitoes, MERS from camels, HIV from primates, and rabies from just about any mammal. In addition, plant pollen, fungi, pet dander, and numerous other substances trigger an immune response (allergic reaction) in susceptible people.

Expensive Nose Hair Threat

What is the easiest way to save a billion dollars in influenza-related healthcare costs? Remind everyone to keep their nose hairs trimmed. While nasal hairs importantly let us know when a bug or dust has been accidentally inhaled, noses usually "itch" for no other reason than the mild irritation created by their hair growing. This causes us to touch our noses many times a day, transferring germs and viruses from every surface and person touched to the interior of the nostrils; in other words, we inoculate ourselves. Of course, the reverse is true, and we pass on our germs to those we care about and everyone else. By trimming your nose hairs, you will decrease your unconscious nose touching, infecting yourself and running up medical costs for everyone.

Biotic stressors increase our stress load and our inflammatory load to some extent, whether they take the form of relatively weak flu viruses the body quickly sweeps away or powerful tuberculosis bacteria the body must wrestle to the mat and destroy over months. Influenza viruses act in a fairly predictable manner, while others, such as the parasite called *Toxoplasmosis gondii*, behave in a much more convoluted way. What follows is a bizarre story about *Toxoplasmosis gondii*, a true story of infection, epigenetics, and behavioral change.

The first item on the list of "Things Mice Fear the Most" is cats. What's the second entry? Cat urine. This fear is so powerful that mice plunge into a panic attack when they smell the stuff. Over the course of millions of years of mouse evolution, they developed a powerful fear of cat urine based on the fact if urine is present, the cat producing it can't be far away. Upon smelling the urine, a mouse will instantly hit the flight button. This increases its chances of surviving long enough to reproduce and pass on the "Cat Urine—RUN!" genes to the next generation: survival of the skittish. These genes are so powerful that laboratory-raised mice exposed to a pad dabbed with cat urine will develop an acute stress reaction and run away, even though they have never seen a cat or smelled its urine before.

In an unexpected plot twist, sometimes mice have the opposite reaction to cat urine: they love it! Whenever they smell it, they look for more and eventually wind up running into a urine-producing cat and committing suicide by feline. Imagine a force powerful enough to entice mice to overcome all those millions of years of evolution to willingly seek out whatever is making that incredible pee.

This suicidal behavior is due to the central nervous system actions of the parasite *Toxoplasmosis gondii,* which life-cycles through its co-hosts in a deadly cat-and-mouse game. A mouse innocently ingests the parasite with its food. This triggers an immune response in the brain, altering the epigenetic response of those cells to such an extent the mouse now pursues cat urine. A cat then eats the mouse, and the *Toxoplasmosis gondii* eggs take up residence in its body, where they hatch and reproduce. New eggs are created and scattered on the ground in the cat's feces until a mouse or a whale or a human ingests them or eats other animals that have ingested them.

No Nobel Here

The discovery of the complete lifecycle of *Toxoplasmosis gondii* was finally proven in 1965. French physicians fed contaminated meat to a group of orphans to see if they developed the classic parasitic brain cysts, and indeed 50 percent did. Nobel Prizes were not awarded for this definitive experiment.

Toxoplasmosis gondii is not just relegated to cats and mice. Humans can also be a host to the parasite if they eat undercooked contaminated meat, consume contaminated water, or come in contact with feces carried on cat paws. Humans are stressed in a different way by *Toxoplasmosis gondii* once it is inside the body. The parasite may settle in the brain and form calcified cysts that cause inflammation in the brain. When pregnant women are exposed to *Toxoplasmosis gondii*, their newborn infants may be born blind. We know some 60 million Americans have been exposed to *Toxoplasmosis gondii*, because their immune systems are producing antibodies designed to destroy the parasite on a second exposure. High levels of these antibodies have been found in the blood of individuals with different types of physical and mental health problems such as dementia, mood disorders, epilepsy, cancer, autoimmune illness, and intestinal disorders.[34]

The antibody response protects humans against future damage from the

---

[34] Jaroslav Flegr, et al, "Toxoplasmosis: A Global Threat. Correlation of Latent Toxoplasmosis with Specific Disease Burden in a Set of 88 Countries," *PLOS ONE 3-24-2014;* https://doi.org/10.1371/journal.pone.0090203.

parasite at the cost of an increase in the inflammatory load from the baseline. In other words, the level of "background inflammation" is higher in these individuals because their immune systems must constantly be a bit more vigilant. (The difference between your resting/normal level of inflammation and the increased level of inflammation caused by any stressor is what I call your *inflammatory load*.)

Kitty Litter

The overproduction of domestic cats has resulted in their feces being swept from the streets into the ocean. Toxoplasmosis has spread to such an extent that antibodies to it have been found in whales and other marine mammals that never come within a thousand miles of inhabited land. Death by this parasite has decimated populations of otters, seals, and sea lions.[35]

Toxoplasmosis gondii is just one example of the many kinds of biotic stressors we wrestle with. Even those stressors not directly causing disease will increase the inflammatory load, eventually contributing to illness and unhealthy aging. Although it would be difficult to calculate how much the inflammatory load rises as new biotic stressors are gradually *added* from the environment, we have seen what happens when these stressors are "suddenly" *removed*. For example, when the British developed their national passion for tea in the late 1700s and began boiling water to prepare the drink, they unintentionally killed harmful bacteria and parasites in the water they previously consumed at room temperature. As the ingestion of biotic stressors dropped, so did the inflammatory load, and the health of the general population improved. This drastic improvement in public health of the eighteenth-century English population made available an excess of healthy workers just as the industrial revolution kicked into gear, enabling England to dominate the world.

Increasing the Biotic Burden

We have long been inadvertently increasing our inflammatory load through exposure to biotic stressors. Perhaps the most common way we do so is through our close contact with animals and other humans. In days past, our ancestors shared their houses with farm animals, and today many of us do the

---

[35] Gloeta Massie, Michael Black, American Society for Microbiology, "Unravelling the Mystery of the Kitty Litter Parasite in Marine Mammals," *Science Daily*, June 5, 2008.

same with pets. Much of the rapidly growing world population lives in large cities, even mega-cities, putting us cheek-to-jowl with many other people and animals, practically all day long. The more we crowd together, sharing germs and wastes, the greater our inflammatory load grows. We can visualize the danger with this simple equation:

$$\uparrow \text{Crowding} \rightarrow \uparrow \text{Biotic/ Psychological Stressors} \rightarrow$$
$$\uparrow \text{Inflammatory Load} \rightarrow \uparrow \text{Illness}$$

Recent bio-archeologic discoveries at the location of one of the first cities in Turkey reveal the breakdown of a civilization due to urbanization. The metropolis started about nine thousand years ago but faded away after a thousand years with evidence of a reduction in the quality of life for those inhabitants as urban living worsened. As population density increased, apartments were crowded close together with evidence of trash pits, dung heaps, and human burials found in many of the interiors. The crowding, along with increasing dependence on grains, took its toll with an increase in poor nutrition, cavities, and infections. It is thought that population density increased aggression in that society because 25 percent of the skeletons found had evidence of healed violent orthopedic injuries.[36]

Another way in which inflammatory load increases is via antibiotic-resistant strains of bacteria. These have evolved in response to the tons of antibiotics given to healthy animals to promote growth and maximize profitability at market at the expense of adverse health consequences to the same customers they are feeding. In recent years, more and more bacteria have become resistant to even our most powerful antibiotics, leading some experts to fear that these new strains will spread through the population. Millions of us could succumb to super-infections that will not be quelled by our immune systems or medicines. Even if we do manage to hold these super bugs at bay, we will suffer tremendously from the increased inflammatory load such an effort will take.

---

[36] Clark Spencer Larsen, et al, "Bioarchaeology of Neolithic Çatalhöyük Reveals Fundamental Transitions in Health, Mobility, and Lifestyle in Early Farmers," *PNAS*, first published June 17, 2019.

The following is a common example of the immune system being overwhelmed, though there is no way to measure the tipping point. The immune system can sequester certain infections within "safe areas" inside the body. The chicken pox (herpes zoster) virus is an example of this. After the acute phase of a chicken pox infection has passed, the virus remains dormant in spinal nerve roots, safely contained by the immune system. However, when the immune response is overwhelmed by other biotic or psychologic stressors, the virus escapes its constraints, replicates, and crawls along the nerves to the skin, where it breaks out as painful viral blisters known as herpes zoster–shingles.

Damage caused by excessive inflammation and an overwhelmed immune system is certainly not a new phenomenon. When scientists examined the blood vessels of Egyptian and Peruvian mummies, they found significant atherosclerosis caused by repeated exposures to tuberculosis, malaria, and other infections.[37] The TB and malaria did not directly attack the arteries; the resulting whole-body inflammation was to blame for eventual death by heart disease or stroke.

Stressors in the Form of Abiotic Challenges: Vitamers to the Rescue

Not only living or "near-living" organisms are harmful; non-living stressors such as chemical toxins, whether natural or artificial, can be just as dangerous. Air pollution, for example, causes immediate irritation and inflammation of the throat and lungs. When severe or in otherwise health-compromised individuals, it can trigger a chronic inflammatory response, with the resulting increase in inflammatory load setting the stage for lung disorders, heart disease, and cancer.[38, 39]

Large-scale exposure to man-made chemicals is a relatively new problem, for just one hundred years ago, people were exposed to relatively few manufactured pollutants. Today, unfortunately, these substances are in and on everything. With the massive increase in industrial chemicals touching all parts of the planet, humanity has entered a terrible new phase in which we begin to suffer toxin exposure *before* birth. For example, in 2017, research showed

---

[37] Gregory S. Thomas, "Why Did Ancient People Have Atherosclerosis? From Autopsies to Computed Tomography to Potential Causes," *Global Heart*, Volume 9, Issue 2, June 2014, 229–237.

[38] Di Ciaula A, et al, "Epigenetic Effects of Air Pollution," *Clinical Handbook of Air Pollution-Related Diseases*, 231–252.

[39] Kyrtopoulos, S., et al, Epigenetic Memory in Response to Environmental Stressors; *FASEB J.*, June 2017, 31(6):2241-2251. doi: 10.1096.

that men exposed to cigarette smoke were more likely to father children with a wide variety of illnesses, even though these fathers were exposed *prior* to conception and not within ninety days of conception. After what we have previously reviewed, it is not surprising that the abiotic toxins in cigarette smoke or air pollution damage sperm through the process of epigenetics.[40]

Once we're born, the onslaught continues, although the damage is not always obvious. A recent study, for instance, found that just two hours of exposure to diesel exhaust can trigger changes at four hundred places on the chromosomes.[41] These changes may later be inherited by children not yet conceived. Unfortunately, although all too aware of their presence, humans do little to protect themselves from abiotic stressors until a significant number of people have been sickened or killed. Think of how long it took to restrict (but not eliminate) cigarette smoking, and how much pollution is still being spewed into the environment.

Some abiotic stressors are known as persistent organic pollutants (POP), because they break down slowly, accumulating in the environment. Dioxin-like chemicals and fire retardants are common POPs. Studies on populations exposed to POPs show that they reduce cellular methylation, resulting in increased risk for all inflammatory illnesses. Finding a population exposed and defined enough to be able to be studied is tricky. This was accomplished in 2008 when researchers examined the Inuit in Greenland. They found higher levels of POPs in the environment, causing lower levels of cellular methylation and leading to greater predisposition to diabetes and heart disease among the Inuit.[42]

Another study, conducted in Korea, came to a similar conclusion when researchers determined that exposure to even low doses of POPs caused direct reductions in methylation levels.[43]

Let's return to a previous example of epigenetic expression to see where the

---

[40]Aston K, et al, "Cigarette Smoking Significantly Alters Sperm DNA Methylation Patterns," *Andrology*, November 2017, 5(6):1089–1099.

[41] Jiang R, Jones MJ, Sava F, et al, "Short-Term Diesel Exhaust Inhalation in a Controlled Human Crossover Study Is Associated with Changes in DNA Methylation of Circulating Mononuclear Cells in Asthmatics," *Particle and Fibre Toxicology*, 2014;11:71.

[42] Rusiecki JS, Baccarelli A, Bollati V, et al, "Global DNA Hypomethylation Is Associated with High Serum-Persistent Organic Pollutants in Greenlandic Inuit," *Environmental Health Perspectives*, 2008; 116:1547–1552.

[43] Kim KY, Kim DS, Lee SK, et al, "Association of Low-Dose Exposure to Persistent Organic Pollutants with Global DNA Hypomethylation in Healthy Koreans," *Environmental Health Perspectives*, 2010; 118(3):370–374.

science of inflammation, vitamers, and epigenetics merge together. Remember the agouti mice, the ones whose babies became sickly yellow butterballs when vitamers were removed from the pregnant mothers' diets? The maternal mice on a normal diet were exposed to a persistent organic pollutant (POP). Their pups, pre-exposed in utero to the previously common chemical toxin bisphenol A (BPA), suffered from hypomethylation similar to what is seen with a folate-deficient diet. The affected mice were obese, yellow-furred, and predisposed to inflammatory diseases of the heart, brain, and endocrine system. The researchers attempted to counteract these detrimental effects by adding additional folate to the mothers' diet. The power of the folate vitamer caused increased methylation, combating abiotic pro-inflammatory stressors and resulting in the birth of normal, healthy mice unaffected by BPA.[44]

Sometimes trying to solve one abiotic stressor problem creates another. Because BPA exposure can set the stage for obesity, cancer, depression, and other ailments, scientists developed a substitute called BPS (bisphenol S). Unfortunately, initial studies suggest BPS might be just as toxic. We cannot currently estimate its effect on health because testing for its pro-inflammatory nature has yet to be fully funded and studied.

Countless Abiotic Stressors, New and Old

A partial list of air and ground contaminants includes carbon monoxide, nitrogen oxides, sulfur dioxides, polycyclic aromatic hydrocarbons, phthalates, formaldehyde, zinc, lead, cadmium, mercury, arsenic, tributyltin, copper, pesticides, methyl parathion, phthalates, dioxins, and polychlorinated biphenyls (PCBs). The Environmental Protection Agency (EPA) has estimated that 2.5 billion pounds of toxic chemicals are released into the environment each year. Many of these chemicals become part of the air pollution so common around the globe, and many of them interfere with the immune response. This results in a wide variety of inflammatory reactions, one of which is linked to the increased frequency of autism in children exposed prior to birth.[45, 46]

---

[44] Dana C Dolinoy, "The Agouti Mouse Model: An Epigenetic Biosensor for Nutritional and Environmental Alterations on the Fetal Epigenome," *Nutrition Reviews*, 2008, 66(Suppl 1):7–11.

[45] Tracy Ann Becerra, et al, "Ambient Air Pollution and Autism in Los Angeles County, California," *Environmental Health Access Perspectives*, Vol. 121, No. 3, March 1, 2013.

[46] Jos Lelieveld, et al, "Cardiovascular Disease Burden from Ambient Air Pollution in Europe Reassessed Using Novel Hazard Ratio Functions," *European Heart Journal*, Volume 40, Issue 20, 21 May 2019, 1590–1596.

You need not be near a source of these substances to be affected, for some are found in the dust blown over from parched, polluted Chinese land spreading around the world on the wind. Then there's the danger from the 600 million pounds of plastics dumped into our oceans every year. Much of this breaks down into microscopic pieces and is eaten by the fish we consume. The increasing concentration of toxins in fish flesh as you move up the food chain is called *bioamplification*.

A new pro-inflammatory threat has arisen in the form of what has been termed *nanopollution*, caused by the increasing demand for the nanotubes necessary for modern manufacturing. Carbon nanotubes are microscopic materials, one ten-thousandth the width of a human hair, used in an increasing number of clothing and consumer products. These nanotubes have been identified in the lungs and white blood cells of children, where they contribute to an inflammatory response manifesting itself as asthma.[47] Some researchers have said the body's inflammatory response to these nanotubes is similar to the response from asbestos exposure, making them highly hazardous substances.

Another source of abiotic stress is the unending parade of new and under-tested chemicals added to our food. Among these are natural and artificial emulsifiers used to enhance taste by helping foods blend together and thicken. These emulsifiers disturb intestinal bacteria, causing an imbalance contributing to an increase in the inflammatory load. Certain emulsifiers have also been linked to increased weight in mice.[48]

Then there are the toxins, allergens, and chemicals brought into our homes by us and our pets without our knowledge or consent. Here's just one way that happens. With people and pets crowded together, we need plenty of flea collars, tick control, and anti-dander treatments. These are necessary, but a study published in *Pediatrics* found low-level indoor insecticides could contribute to an increased risk of childhood leukemia, lymphoma, and brain tumors.[49] The EPA's attempts to regulate and reduce exposure to these toxins have been hamstrung by lobbyists and members of Congress, meaning that many pesticides that have been outlawed as dangerous toxins in other countries are still allowed here. The situation is only getting worse.

---

[47] Kolosnjaj-Tabi J, Just J, Hartman KB, et al, "Anthropogenic Carbon Nanotubes Found in the Airways of Parisian Children," *EBioMedicine*, 2015, 2(11):1697–1704.
[48] Chassaing B, Gewirtz AT, "Dietary Emulsifiers Impact the Mouse Gut Microbiota Promoting Colitis and Metabolic Syndrome, *Nature*, 2015, 519:92–96.
[49] Chen, M, Chang CH, Tao L, Lu C., "Residential Exposure to Pesticide During Childhood and Childhood Cancers: A Meta-Analysis," *Pediatrics*, 2015, 136(4):719–729.

Abiotics, Obesity, and Infertility

I mentioned earlier that certain emulsifiers have been linked to increased weight gain in mice. This is not a random finding, nor a surprising one, for many of these additives have been found to interfere with normal homeostatic functions. Some of these chemicals, known as endocrine disruptors, fool the hormonal system by mimicking the body's naturally produced hormones. Posing as real hormones, these substances upset homeostasis in one of two ways. They can stimulate hormonal receptors to produce too much of a hormone response, or they can block the receptors where hormones normally "plug in," preventing any benefits of naturally produced hormones. Depending on which hormone functions are disrupted, the consequences range from mild to serious and include male and female infertility, thyroid abnormalities, childhood developmental problems, and mood dysfunction.

Another new source of abiotic toxin exposure comes from chemicals used to extract certain energy sources through the environmentally dangerous practice of fracking. These chemicals disrupt the endocrine system and are linked to the emergence of fertility problems in oil field workers with prenatal abnormalities in their offspring.[50] I guess it's just the cost of doing business someone else is paying for with their health, future fertility, and lagging childhood development in their exposed children.

Obeying Obesogens

Between the environment, natural and man-made chemicals, viruses, bacteria, and more, we're being hit from every direction by biotic and abiotic stressors. Ecotoxicology researchers have investigated the effects of abiotic and biotic stressors and come to the disturbing conclusions these disruptors can also be agents encouraging obesity (obesogens.) These obesogenic endocrine disruptors work by triggering abnormalities in the way the body manufactures and stores fat.[51] For example, it has been suggested one cause of the worldwide obesity epidemic might be inflammation caused by exposure to chemical toxins. The problem is certainly more complex

[50] Nagel SN, "Developmental and Reproductive Effects of Chemicals Associated with Unconventional Oil and Natural Gas Operations," *Reviews on Environmental Health*, 2014, 29(4):307–318.

[51]Grug F., Blumberg B., "Endocrine Disrupters as Obesogens," *Molecular and Cellular Endocrinology*, 2009, 304(1-2):19–29.

than just overeating or a sedentary lifestyle.[52] Of course, there are secondary effects, for few health problems fail to trigger other problems. For example, increased weight in males is associated with decreased fertility, and excess adipose tissue in general is linked to inflammation and heart disease. If we put this into an equation, it would be:

$$\text{Toxins} \rightarrow \uparrow \text{Inflammatory Response} \rightarrow \uparrow \text{Adipose Tissue} \rightarrow \uparrow \text{Diabetes/Heart Disease}$$

Various biotic and abiotic toxins may be working directly on the cell, creating an inflammatory response and cell death. They also may be reducing DNA-methylation, resulting in pro-inflammatory consequences. Hypomethylation caused by abiotic toxin compounds, combined with hypomethylation caused by inadequate nutrition and vitamer intake, significantly raises the risk of serious health consequences. This deadly combination is most likely the basis for most of our current medical difficulties.[53]

Climate Change and Stress

Changes in the environment have always been one of the major long-term stressors for all living organisms. As human activity causes accelerated climate change, more people will be stressed by temperature extremes, water shortages, nutrient deficiency, and resulting emotional stress. In addition, the more energy used to heat or cool ourselves from these extremes, and the more we rely on energy and chemicals to produce and transport our food and water, the more toxins we are exposed to, increasing our inflammatory loads. The connection between climate change as a stressor and the change it makes in our epigenetic makeup is a new field of research called *environmental epigenetics*. This important area of research will ultimately determine how we survive into the future.

Adding to the Burden

Even as we're adding to our inflammatory burden, processed food

---

[52] Baillie-Hamilton, P.F., "Chemical Toxins: A Hypothesis to Explain the Global Obesity Epidemic," *Journal of Alternative and Complementary Medicine*, 2002, 8(2):185–192.

[53] Lee, D.H., Jacobs, D.R., Porta, M., "Hypothesis: A Unifying Mechanism for Nutrition and Chemicals as Lifelong Modulators of DNA Hypomethylation," *Environmental Health Perspectives*, 2009, 117(12):1799–1802.

manufacturing is subtracting the nutrients needed to combat inflammation. The manufacturers often try to compensate by adding back inferior forms of vital nutrients. Folic acid instead of folate is one example. This double whammy is worsened through reliance on modern medications, many of which reduce B12 and folate levels in the body. These medicines include metformin, prescribed to diabetics to lower blood sugar.[54]

Lowering elevated blood sugar is beneficial, but metformin blocks B12 and folate, which worsens diabetic peripheral neuropathy and cardiovascular disease. Among the other medications lowering B12 and folate levels are antibiotics, anticonvulsants, nicotine, neomycin, proton pump inhibitors like omeprazole, H-2 antagonists like ranitidine and cimetidine, nitrous oxide, male and female hormone replacement therapy, and birth control pills.

From Abiotic to Biotic

As mentioned, climate change is forcing us to seek new sources of heat, food, and water as an abiotic stress. Unfortunately, climate change also spawns biotic stress. A large number of viruses, bacteria, and parasites reside in South and Central America, preferring the warmer temperatures in those areas. As other areas of the globe warm up, these dangers can spread. The Zika virus is just one of many moving into the Northern Hemisphere, transmitted by the same mosquito spreading yellow fever. Zika interferes with development of the fetal nervous system, causing babies to be born with smaller-than-normal brains. (Does this virus affect the epigenetics of brain development?) This one of the many "climate change infections" we are now forced to deal with.

Stressors in Psychological Form

The third kind of stressors are psychological in nature. They arise within the brain and are the most complex of all. Psychological stress is less tangible, for it does not come to us in the form of cells or molecules or something else we can identify and measure. Instead, psychological stress "enters" the brain

---

[54] Xu, L., Huang, Z., He, X., et al, "Adverse Effect of Metformin Therapy on Serum Vitamin B12 and Folate: Short-Term Treatment Causes Disadvantages?" *Medical Hypotheses*, 2013; 81(2):149–51.

invisibly via what we see, hear, feel, taste, or smell. Psychological stressors are often first identified when someone develops clinical symptoms associated with depression, anxiety, and other emotional illnesses.

One morning during my college summer break, I had just arrived home from my job as an orderly at Norfolk General Hospital. I remember being famished, having just prepared my meal before hearing the phone ring. That call changed my life, yet other than holding the receiver to my ear, nothing physically touched me. Words had been converted into electrical energy, transmitted and turned back into the physical energy of sound waves from the phone's vibrating speaker. But the force of the words was so great that my body reacted physically. It was as though I had been in a violent car crash. Alarm signals rang through my sympathetic nervous system, overwhelming my brain as it tried to make sense of awful words I was hearing. These signals instructed my system to dump out copious amounts of adrenaline, causing a hot rush to burn through my body. My heart raced, my breathing accelerated, and the blood vessels near my skin constricted, making me feel clammy. I'm sure my face turned pale in color. My appetite disappeared instantly, replaced by nausea as I angrily shoved my plate away and began to sob.

That phone call triggered an inflammatory response, instantaneously and system-wide. I looked and felt ill, and over the next week, I developed the classic "sickness behaviors" of fatigue, depression, poor sleep, reduced appetite, and anhedonia. My body behaved as though it were in a death struggle, putting out strong inflammatory proteins in response, but there were no invaders or physical wounds, no car crash, only those words I had heard coming through the phone from the very hospital I had left: "Your brother was admitted earlier today and just died." This emotional assault was more painful than any physical one I had ever or would ever experience. The resulting intermittent episodes of anxiety and depression continued for years, intensifying my inflammatory load and over time contributing to my own health predispositions.

Unforgiving Living

Emotional interaction with other humans—living, loving, and losing—are hardwired into our genes. We are made to live in moderate-sized communities with other humans, which is why solitary confinement for extended periods of time is considered to be such a cruel punishment. We are social animals, but unfortunately our social, physical, and emotional evolution has not prepared us to thrive in the overwhelming, overcrowded communities of modern life.

The number of large urban locales has exploded in the seventy-some years since World War II. Extensive protein, folate, and B12 transport (meat and vegetables) permitted by superior refrigeration, combined with advances in building materials, has allowed an explosion of dense stressful urban living assemblies all over the world—unforgiving living. Unfortunately, because of this density we often have little control over interpersonal distance, and this lack of control is one of the greatest sources of psychological stress. When you put too many people too close together, with few options to find "space," some of them erupt with expressions of anger, depression, and anxiety.

Having plenty of control over individual social space made early America unique, and people sought it out. Some of the lands they came from had less food, water, or space. Ours was a large country, and the cost of moving on down the road to a less crowded place was relatively small. Living in America once allowed you to choose your relational distances, which helped reduce anxiety, but that perk is being lost. Interpersonal distance is becoming more and more expensive, and options for self-reliance are becoming limited, increasing our collective inflammatory load.

And so, there is a quandary. We are genetically wired to interact with others, but too much forced interaction increases the risk of emotional stress and inflammation. This increase in inflammation due to interpersonal stress can be found in adults who were bullied as children. In those individuals, the markers of inflammation were found to be just as great as those of children who had been physically abused and neglected by their parents.[55]

In 1967, psychiatrists Thomas Holmes and Richard Rahe developed the "Life Change Index Scale" as a way of measuring the amount of psychological stress one might be carrying. It's not a measure of the stress itself or of the changes in the level of inflammation within the body. Instead, it's a way of converting common life events into a numerical total suggesting the odds of developing a stress-related breakdown in physical health.

The scale, commonly called the Holmes Scale, assigns points to most of the psychological stressors occurring in life, including divorce, death in the family, illness, injury, financial problems, work concerns, moving, sleep changes, and legal difficulties. The higher the point total, the greater the risk of developing physical and emotional symptoms of chronic stress, such as headaches, elevated blood pressure, increased heart rate, intestinal upset, muscle tension,

---

[55] Copeland, W.E., Wolke, D., Lereya, S. T., et al, "Childhood Bullying Involvement Predicts Low-Grade Systemic Inflammation into Adulthood," *Proceedings of the National Academy of Sciences of the United States of America*, 2014, 111(21):7570–7575.

fatigue, depression, anxiety, poor self-esteem, sleep difficulty, and attention difficulties. We know there is an association between these manifestations and an increase in inflammatory markers. For example, when these stressors cause poor sleep or a reduction in physical activity— the most common expressions of psychological stress—the inflammatory response is exacerbated.[56]

Mind and body are intimately linked; indeed, they are really one and the same, different aspects of the whole person. The brain is not separate from the body; what happens in one is always reflected in what happens in the other, in reciprocal fashion.

Measuring Stress by Monitoring Inflammation

There is a way to "look" inside the body and see if it is being assaulted by stress. It's not perfect, but it gives us an indication of what may lie ahead.

When biotic, abiotic, or psychological stressors trigger an inflammatory response, fat cells and macrophage white blood cells begin churning out cytokines. When these protein messengers reach the liver, they signal the hepatic cells to make numerous defensive proteins, one of which is called C-reactive protein (CRP). In equation form, it looks like this:

$$\text{Stressor} \rightarrow \text{Inflammatory Response} \rightarrow \text{Cytokine Release} \rightarrow \text{Liver} \rightarrow \text{CRP Release}$$

CRP floods the bloodstream, preparing to deal with the result of injury or illness by breaking up weakened or dying human cells. This is part of the inflammatory response that prepares the body to extinguish foreign assailants, destroy damaged cells, and repair and renew other cells. CRP levels can be easily measured in a blood sample, with a higher number indicating an increase in the degree of inflammatory response. While this blood test offers an indication of the degree and eventual resolution of inflammation, there is such variability between stressors and individual responses that its practical applications are limited. Other laboratory tests (see chapter twelve) are better able to measure the body's inflammatory response to a stressor, but they require special equipment and procedures, making it beyond the reach of

---

[56] Bernert, R.A., Turvey, C.L., Conwell, Y., Joiner, T.E., "Association of Poor Subjective Sleep Quality with Risk for Death by Suicide During a 10-Year Period: A Longitudinal, Population-Based Study of Late Life, *JAMA Psychiatry*, 2014; 71(10):1129–37.

clinical practice. For now, we can use CRP levels and white blood cell levels, which rise when the body mounts a stress response, to get a general sense of the body's inflammation load.

There are many situations and illnesses that elevate CRP, the most common being excess adipose (fat) tissue. The greater the adipose tissue mass, the higher the inflammatory load and baseline CRP level. This simply means that being overweight is a source of inflammation and stress. Other causes for elevated CRP levels include cigarette smoking, high blood pressure, prescription hormones, gum disease, arthritis, cancer, diabetes, pregnancy, burns, excessive exercise, and natural aging. Factors lowering inflammation and CRP levels include moderate exercise and a reduction in fat tissue, whether through weight loss or surgery. Many studies have shown a reduction in pro-inflammatory proteins after gastric bypass surgery weight loss.[57]

With a more precise test known as high-sensitivity CRP (hs-CRP), physicians can track the progression of an acute inflammation-related illness like a heart attack, watching as the level rises and falls before and during treatment. The greater the challenge, the higher the CRP level in the blood. For a severe, whole-body infection, it can shoot up by more than forty thousand times in just two days!

CRP levels vary from person to person, making it difficult to look at a single, moderately high reading and say whether it is good or bad. For this reason, some people like to have their CRP level tested to establish a baseline. If you decide to do so, be sure you are free of illness, injury, or infection when tested so you'll have a true reading. Always remember that the increase in inflammatory load caused by any stressor varies from person to person, so it is not yet possible to use CRP as the ultimate guide to health and disease. Fortunately, medical science is marching ahead, and soon, when more specific testing is available, we will be able to track the inflammatory course of numerous diseases and specifically determine how much B12 and folate vitamers can assist in reducing inflammatory load.

Someday, we may even have a way to measure an ongoing inflammatory process in real time without the need for blood tests. Cells under stress shrink and have more extracellular water around them, affecting the speed (impedance) at which an electrical current moves through tissues. Dr. Tsigos and colleagues measured this impedance via sensors on the skin and say that this technology "may provide a useful, bloodless and rapid tool in the clinical

---

[57] Catalán, V., "Proinflammatory Cytokines in Obesity: Impact of Type 2 Diabetes Mellitus and Gastric Bypass Obesity," *Surgery*, 2007; 17(11):1464–1474.

setting, distinguishing patients with chronic stress/inflammation from healthy subjects and monitoring their response to treatment."[58]

Compounded Stressors

Now that we have looked at the three kinds of stressors, we can look at a contemporary scenario of how they can be connected to each other in a series of events. The abiotic stress of climate change is causing the level of CO_2 in our air to go up. This leads to inferior crop production because the stressed plants cannot make as many essential proteins and other nutrients.[17] This creates the biotic stressor of decreased nutrient intake for consumers. Subsistence farmers and their families suffer the psychologic stressor of food and economic insecurity.

The Universal Illness

In review, there are biotic, abiotic, and psychological stressors causing stress reactions presenting as symptoms of chronic inflammation. Inflammation, whether chronic or acute, is the foundation for almost all illnesses and for this reason should be called the Universal Illness.

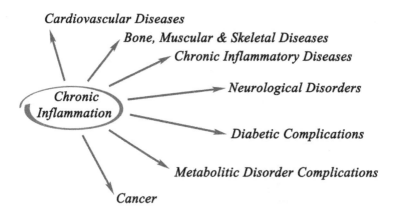

[58] Tsigos, C., Stefanaki, C., Lambrou, G.I., Boschiero, D., Chrousos, G.P., "Stress and Inflammatory Biomarkers and Symptoms Are Associated with Bioimpedance Measures, *European Journal of Clinical Investigation*, 2015; 45(2):126–34.

Next Up: Modulating the Stress Response

The relationship between the stress response and disease is affected by the nature, number, and persistence of the stressors, as well as by an individual's biological and emotional vulnerability. In the next chapter, we will take a half-step back in our equations to add two new concepts I refer to as your unique biological and psychological vulnerability—your lens and how you can modulate the expression of stress coming through your lens. Very simply, a lens is an entity that focuses or diffuses incoming stressors. We will discuss the factors making up this lens of vulnerability and the various modulators available that can be integrated to reduce your inflammatory load. Guess which one is the most important modulator?

EIGHT

LENSES AND MODULATORS

(lens)

Stressor→⬛→Healthy Modulation→↓Stress Response→
↓Illness→↑Healthy Longevity

Forty-year-old Dianne had just completed her late-afternoon 10K run. As a competitive triathlete, she took her training seriously, never missing a day. She felt good after that day's workout despite the dry Southern California Santa Ana winds sucking much of the moisture out of the air. Dianne breezed into her kitchen, where the children worked on their homework at the dining room table. She had just begun to prepare dinner when she collapsed on the floor with a massive, fatal heart attack.

How could that have happened? Don't women have some genetic "protection" against heart attacks, at least until after menopause? And aren't people who throw themselves into intensive aerobic exercise—including the running, swimming, and bicycling required of a triathlete—supposed to be nearly immune to cardiovascular disease?

Yes, and yes. Premenopausal women are less likely to suffer heart attacks than men of the same age, and regular aerobic exercise does indeed help ward off clogged arteries. What really mattered in this case were the factors protecting Dianne from, and predisposing her to, a heart attack. To understand these, we must stop thinking of Dianne as a statistic, part of a large group, and examine her up close, as a single and unique person. In other words, we must look at her unique lens, her one-of-a-kind blend of genetics, epigenetics, diet, and medications in place and influencing her mind and body up until the time the last stressor overwhelmed her. Afterward, we will consider the ways she might have positively modulated her body's stress response toward a more fortuitous outcome.

As it happened, those dry Santa Ana winds sucked moisture out of everything, including Dianne, causing dehydration. Her high-intensity exercise regimen produced more dehydration with an increase in muscle cell damage, further increasing her inflammatory load. (While exercise is necessary for good health, too much can lead to low-level chronic muscle inflammation.) Dianne also took birth control pills, which are known to prevent the conversion of the vitamin folic acid into bioavailable folate.[59] The reduction of folate caused a significant increase in the levels of the cellular waste product homocysteine, which caused her blood to thicken— increased viscosity. These three factors—dehydration, chronic inflammation, and elevated homocysteine—caused a dangerous thickening of her blood. In the end, it was not surprising that a blood clot formed and triggered a fatal heart attack. In equation form, the "story" of Dianne's lens and modulators looks like this:

$$\text{Birth Control Pills} + \text{Dehydration} + \text{Chronic Inflammation} \rightarrow$$
$$\downarrow\text{Folate} \rightarrow \uparrow\text{Homocysteine} \rightarrow \uparrow\text{Blood Viscosity} \rightarrow$$
$$\uparrow\text{Clots} \rightarrow \text{Heart Attack}$$

For Dianne, this was a fatal equation. For other people, it is not. Their bodies might be better at absorbing vitamers from food, holding on to fluids, tamping down inflammation, cleaning up excessive homocysteine, or doing any number of other things allowing them to do exactly what Dianne did that day, without the fatal heart attack. Then again, they may be struck by a problem that would leave Dianne unscathed, for everyone has a distinctive lens made up of multiple factors, some able to be modulated and some not. For example, a simple modulation she could have initiated was to consider the dry weather conditions and hyper-hydrate before, during, and after her normal routine.

---

[59] Wakeman, Michael P., "A Review of the Effects of Oral Contraceptives on Nutrient Status, with Especial Consideration to Folate in UK," *Journal of Advances in Medicine and Medical Research*, July 11, 2019.

Athletic Risks–Sudden Athletics Cessation Syndrome

The risk for developing blood clots worsens with any one of the following: being vegan, having a sudden decrease or increase in athletics, or a new pregnancy. All of those individually increase the cellular waste product homocysteine, causing the blood to thicken and increasing the likelihood of clot (embolus) formation.

Let's say there was an incredible hard-driving female athlete, a vegan, at the top of her physical condition with a significant positive muscle mass due to her peak performance. Then there is a sudden reduction in her physical activity and muscle stimulation because of an injury or a newly discovered pregnancy. I call this Sudden Athletics Cessation Syndrome. Excess muscle protein must be broken down because the body is told that it is no longer needed. If you are involved in intense physical activity, the muscle protein can break down the same way it does from an injury. These real-life situations will increase the amino acid homocysteine, bringing about thickening of the blood. B12 and folate vitamers are required to break down this waste product to reduce the risk of roaming blood clots. Being vegan, pregnant, suddenly inactive, or any combination of these make reducing homocysteine all that much harder.[60] (Creating a whole new human being during pregnancy requires a lot of extra B12 and folate vitamers that are transferred away from the mother to the developing fetus, particularly in the first trimester.)

Adjusting Your Lens

Your response to stressors, disrupted homeostasis, and inflammation are fixed to some degree by your genes. And you can't alter your genes, because you can't change your parents, but you can change the way many of your genes are expressed—your "epigenetic line-up"—as well as hundreds of other factors that may help promote or alleviate inflammation. It helps to think of this ability to alter the way your body responds to stressors—indeed, to everything in its environment—in terms of *lenses* and *modulators*.

Your *lens* consists of everything you are, right at this very moment: your genetic inheritance and epigenetics. These factors and more act as the lens

---

[60] Burkert, N.T., et al, "The Association between Eating Behavior and Various Health Parameters," *Nutrition and Health*, 2014, PloS ONE 9(2): e88278 doi:10.1371.

through which stressors are processed. That's why an identical stressor strikes two people simultaneously yet produce very different effects. One person may be genetically predisposed to having strong, thick bones, while another has inherited a tendency toward fragile, thin bones. When each takes a similar tumble off a bicycle, one walks away unscathed, while the other suffers a broken bone. While this is a simple example, the interplay between your lens and your reactions to stressors is often more subtle and complex, yet the concept remains the same.

Modulators include all the things you do to "adjust" your stress response—in other words, to produce a more positive or less negative response to a stressor. A change in diet or exercise habits can be a modulator, as can spending more time with friends and family. Even something as seemingly minor as cutting back on soda consumption can be a modulator.

Modulators can be utilized to adjust your lens in two ways: before the stressor hits and after. You can exercise and lose weight if you are at risk of a heart attack, thus making your lens more efficient in processing any significant additional stressor. Let's say you did have a heart attack; you can use the same modulators—exercise and weight control—more consistently, plus you can add modulators to reduce the stress response to the next stressor coming through. Your lens is never static, as you are always making positive or negative adjustments consciously or unconsciously. This dynamic will be explained more clearly in diagrammatic form when we graph some of the ways stressors and modulators are processed over time in chapter twelve.

Here is a list of the most common modulators affecting our lives positively or negatively:

- dietary intake
- caffeine intake
- level of social connectivity
- medications
- supplements
- sleep habits
- air pollution
- emotional response to events
- meditation
- amount and type of exercise

- toxins eaten, inhaled, touched
- family relationships
- vitamer intake

It would be impossible to list all the potential positive and negative modulators; instead, we'll look at few easy positive ones that make big improvements in your health.

Vitamers as Modulators

As we've discussed, increasing blood levels of vitamer B12 and folate is one of the most important modulations you can make. While your genetics are fixed, your levels of these vitamers are not, giving you the opportunity to bring them up to optimal and keeping them there. And as we have also discussed, B12 and folate are particularly important modulators, influencing everything from red blood cell production to the manufacturing of neurotransmitters, from homocysteine reduction to the maintenance of healthy low inflammatory homeostasis. None of the other modulators—exercise, meditation, reduced carbohydrate intake, etc.—work optimally unless ample supplies of B vitamers are available.

This is because B12 and folate are "rate-limiters" of biochemical reactions. That is, a deficiency of either acts as a restraint on the cellular processes, making the reactions less efficient. Let's map it out. Suppose you begin with a certain amount of substrate. With the assistance of cofactors, in this case B12/F, a chemical substrate will be converted into an end-product. When 100 percent of the required B12/F is available, the process will be very efficient, producing close to 100 percent of the final product.

$$\text{Cofactors B}_{12}/\text{F (100\%)}$$
$$\downarrow$$
$$\text{Substrate (100\%)} \rightarrow \text{Final Product (100\%)}$$

Suppose only half of the required amount of B12/F is available. Even though you begin with the same amount of substrate as in the previous equation, the process will be inefficient. Fifty percent of the substrate will not be acted on, yielding only 50 percent of the final product.

Co-factors B12/F (50%)

↓

Substrate (100%) → Final Product (50%)

In the language of the cell, this means that you will only have half of the cellular energy production you might otherwise have: half of the reduction in homocysteine, half the DNA methylation, and so much more. This "half-itis" triggers a bewildering variety of problems, including depression, anxiety, fatigue, cardiovascular symptoms, weight gain, poor wound healing, and gastrointestinal disturbance. And because these sorts of problems are often complex and caused by a variety of factors, identifying a deficiency as part of the illness is usually a low priority.

A small number of health professionals are beginning to consider the role of B12 and folate vitamers in depression and other forms of emotional distress, thanks to papers appearing in the medical literature. A 2010 article described what happened when a twenty-nine-year-old patient with a long history of depressive symptoms was treated with antidepressants.[61] The first medication did not work, so he was given a second, then a third. Only after three failures was a more detailed personal history taken, revealing that the patient maintained a vegan diet. Further lab tests were then ordered, which showed that the patient had a low B12 blood level. When he was given vitamers B12 and folate in addition to an antidepressant, his depression resolved, as did his physical symptoms. He continued taking the antidepressant and vitamers and remained symptom-free thereafter—*nutritional psychiatry*.

I made this same mistake with my patients; trying one antidepressant after another without considering B12/folate levels. Once I learned about vitamers, I began asking my patients about the kinds and amounts of meat they were eating and the types of supplements they were taking. If there was any indication that they might be low in vitamers, I investigated further.

B12 and folate are not a cure-all; they're the foundation keeping your biochemical machinery churning at its most efficient speed.

We'll take a more in-depth look at the relationship between vitamers and inflammation in the next chapter.

---

[61] Kate, N., Grover, S., Agarwal, M., "Does B12 Deficiency Lead to Lack of Treatment Response to Conventional Antidepressants?" *Psychiatry* (Edgmont), 2010; 7(11):42–44.

Exercise Prize

Assuming you are taking in adequate amounts of the vitamers and other nutrients, exercise is a powerful positive modulator. That's because moderate—not excessive—exercise increases muscle energy production, reduces inflammation, and prompts positive epigenetic changes in the way fat is stored by improving methylation.[62] These cells become better at producing energy, and the body's ability to use insulin to regulate glucose levels is improved, helping ward off diabetes. Of course, if you do not have enough vitamers to "fund" the methylation, you cannot enjoy the full benefits of exercise.

Physical workouts in moderation exert anti-inflammatory effects by increasing the levels of myokines, one of the many hundreds of cytokines produced and released by muscle cell contraction. Myokines trigger epigenetic changes that help adipose cells metabolize more efficiently, thus reducing body fat. Excessive fat tissue uses up folate and are pro-inflammatory in and of themselves,[63] while the myokines help to tamp down long-term inflammation.[64] Conversely, a decrease in daily movement that occurs with a desk job requiring extensive sitting is associated with increased inflammation.

The anti-inflammatory effects of exercise also help the brain by increasing blood flow and the production of neurotransmitters.[65] Exercise plus B12 and folate vitamers increase communication between brain cells by helping neural connections grow. This improves cognitive function and reduces the development of cellular changes seen in Alzheimer's disease.

Fortunately, exercise is an easy modulator to adopt, and you can get started with simple brisk walking. If you do nothing more than go from being a couch potato to a regular walker, it's an improvement. The addition of resistance training can do even more to reduce inflammation in your brain and body.

---

[62] Rönn, T., Volkov, P., Davegardh, C., et al, "A Six Months Exercise Intervention Influences the Genome-Wide DNA Methylation Pattern in Human Adipose Tissue, *PLoS Genetics*, 2013; 9(6):e1003572.

[63] Mahabir, S., Ettinger, S., Johnson, L., Baer, D.J., Clevidence, B.A., Hartman, T.J., Taylor, P.R., "Measures of Adiposity and Body Fat Distribution in Relation to Serum Folate Levels in Postmenopausal Women in a Feeding Study." *Eur J Clin Nutr.*, May 2008; 62(5):644–50.

[64] Benatti, F.B., Pedersen, B.K., "Exercise as an Anti-Inflammatory Therapy for Rheumatic Diseases—Myokine Regulation," *Nature Reviews Rheumatology*, 2015, 11:86–97.

[65] Cotman, C.W., Berchtold, N.C., Christie, L.A. "Exercise Builds Brain Health: Key Roles of Growth Factor Cascades and Inflammation," *Cell*, 2007; 30(9):464–472.

Knees' Needs

If you consider exercise to be one of the most important tools in your toolbox, to be used every day for the rest of your life, then the foundation of that modulator is your knees. Start protecting them as early in life as possible. When they start to hurt on a regular basis after a workout, damage has most likely started. One way to protect them is to limit walking down stairs and steep hills when you have a choice. When walking up, many muscles and tendons stabilize the knee, but going down there are fewer, which we intuitively know because going up is always more tiring than going down.

To protect your knees, consciously activate your leg muscles before contact rather than letting the muscles unconsciously contract after contact and knee-joint pressure has occurred. Our knees were not made to go down stairs in regular steps for very long because this was not a survival tool needed on the savannah. One way to reduce pressure is to walk downhill with shorter, bended-knee steps or touch the ground with your toe first as when you run downhill. When going down stairs, use your arms on the railing to reduce pressure on knees. Though this technique takes active attention to what your leg muscles are communicating, it is worth the benefits of better weight and mood control for the rest of your life.

In some cases, however, exercise is a negative modulator. It is possible to exercise too vigorously, causing stress on all the body's cells, muscle protein breakdown, and a rise in homocysteine levels. The body cannot handle this, even with adequate B_{12}/F levels. Homocysteine levels rise with excess exercise because of the increased workload on all body cells, resulting in more muscle damage and waste production. Increased homocysteine by itself may lead to inflammation and nerve damage.[66]

Sleep Upkeep

Adequate sleep is necessary for inflammation control, the maintenance of a vigorous immune system, and brain health.[67] The pro-inflammatory

---

[66] Xiaojie Zhang, "Folic Acid Protects Motor Neurons against the Increased Homocysteine, Inflammation and Apoptosis in SOD1 Transgenic Mice," *Neuropharmacology*, June 2008, 54(7):1112–9.

[67] Janet M. Mullington, Ph.D., et al, "Sleep Loss and Inflammation," *Best Pract Res Clin Endocrinol Metab*, October 2010; 24(5):775–784.

effects of too little sleep were demonstrated in a 2013 study in which one group of healthy volunteers was restricted to four hours of sleep a night for five nights, while a comparison group was allowed eight hours.[68] The results were alarming: sleep restriction altered the expression of 117 genes, including some regulating the immune system. The researchers noted that some of the gene alterations "appear to be long-lasting and may at least partially explain how prolonged sleep restriction contributes to inflammation-associated pathological states, such as cardiometabolic diseases."

A 2012 study illustrated the association between sleep deprivation and the immune response.[69] The researchers gave subjects vaccinations against hepatitis B and then measured their antibody responses over time—in other words, they looked at how well the vaccination was "taking." They found that those who got less sleep had significantly reduced responses to their vaccinations, producing fewer of the desired antibody proteins.

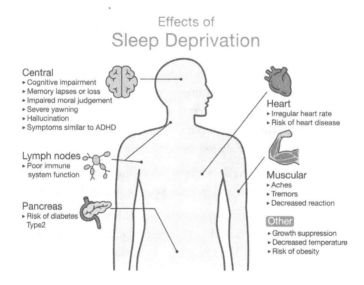

Effects of
Sleep Deprivation

Central
- Cognitive impairment
- Memory lapses or loss
- Impaired moral judgement
- Severe yawning
- Hallucination
- Symptoms similar to ADHD

Lymph nodes
- Poor immune system function

Pancreas
- Risk of diabetes Type2

Heart
- Irregular heart rate
- Risk of heart disease

Muscular
- Aches
- Tremors
- Decreased reaction

Other
- Growth suppression
- Decreased temperature
- Risk of obesity

There is also a clear connection between getting adequate sleep and maintaining brain health. During sleep, brain cells actually shrink, with the space between them increasing by up to 60 percent. This allows more

[68] Aho, V., Ollila, H. M., Rantanen, V., et al, "Partial Sleep Restriction Activates Immune Response-Related Gene Expression Pathways: Experimental and Epidemiological Studies in Humans," *PLoS ONE*, 2013; 8(10): e77184. doi:10.1371/journal.pone.0077184.

[69] Prather, A.A., Hall, M., Fury, J.M., et al, "Sleep and Antibody Response to Hepatitis B Vaccination," *Sleep*, 2012; 35(8):1063–1069.

cerebrospinal fluid to circulate. This increased circulation improves the ability of the brain's waste-disposal system (the glymphatic system) to remove dead cells, waste products building up during waking hours, and plaque-producing chemicals associated with Alzheimer's disease.[70]

While the ideal amount of sleep varies from person to person, most people don't get sufficient amounts of restorative sleep, the normal sleep cycle that allows you to awake refreshed and fully able to function. Here are a few tips to help you get ample amounts of restorative sleep:

- Don't underestimate the amount of sleep you need. If you have trouble remaining focused during the day, if you need caffeine later in the day for a pickup, if you find your energy level falling—you're probably not getting enough restorative sleep.

- Don't try to be a "hero" by working into your sleeping hours.

- Respect your natural rhythms. Your body produces hormones like serotonin and melatonin at specific times each day to wake you up and prepare you for sleep. You help this natural cycle by going to bed and getting up at the same time every day, even on weekends. When you stay up late on Saturday night, you'll want to sleep in on Sunday morning, and you then may find it hard to go to sleep at your regular time on Sunday night (a condition known as "Sunday night insomnia"). This makes it extra hard to get up on Monday morning feeling rested and ready for the week ahead.

- Avoid eating or exercise late into the evening, as both activities ramp up your metabolism and increase your "wake-up hormones."

- Reduce your exposure to electronic light for an hour or so before going to bed, especially blue (daylight) wavelengths that stimulate brain wakefulness. You can purchase inexpensive glasses with lenses that filter out blue wavelengths, use light-altering software, or simply turn off electronic devices, including the television, well before bedtime.

- Keep your bedroom as cool as possible. Each partner should arrange his or her own temperature control zones with their own layers of clothing and blankets. Sleep cycles are disrupted by comforters and nightclothes kept on too long after the weather

---

[70] Frank, M.G., "The Role of Glia in Sleep Regulation and Function," *Handb Exp Pharmacol*, 2019; 253:83–96.

starts to warm up in the spring. (Personal tip: Using two top sheets, one of which can be folded back if the temperature increases, often give better temperature control than one blanket.)

- Elevate the head of your bed by placing the two-inch side of a two-by-four block under the head-end legs. Uneven floors combine with uneven bed frames, worn mattresses, and the extra weight of the upper body to make your head lie a few degrees lower than your legs. Sleeping with your head lower increases the risk of developing sleep apnea, snoring, and ear infections as well as gastric reflux because of the downward pressure on the esophageal sphincter. This reflux is then treated with PPIs or H2s which decreases B_{12}/F.

Reducing Ear Infections–An Old Pediatric Trick

One simple technique I learned in my training from an older pediatrician is to have parents slightly elevate the head of their child's bed with these simple wooden blocks. This helps prevent the pooling of secretions or recently fed milk near the inner ear opening in the back of the throat. This also diminishes GERD symptoms, reducing the need for PPIs and H2 inhibitors in children. Wood blocks could save a billion dollars in healthcare costs, reducing the need for repeated antibiotic treatments, surgical interventions, and future hearing disabilities.

Anxiety Reduction as Modulator

Stressors, physical or emotional, reduce the body's ability to maintain homeostasis and, therefore, optimal health. One way stress does this is by increasing the production of pro-inflammatory cytokines in the body.[71] This, along with other stress-induced changes, hampers the body's ability to fight infections, other pathogens, and the proliferation of cancer cells. As chronic stress builds, the body's capacity to adjust and maintain homeostasis becomes

---

[71] Maes, M., "The Effects of Psychological Stress on Humans: Increased Production of Pro-Inflammatory Cytokines and Th1-Like Response in Stress-Induced Anxiety," *Cytokine*, 1998; 19(4):313–318.

hampered, leading to the inflammatory diseases of chronic heart disease, asthma, and many other ailments.[72]

Let's look at emotional stress, in the form of anxiety, an omnipresent aspect of the human condition. Well before the development of spoken language, we knew life was fraught with danger. We weren't nearly as fast, strong, or sharp-toothed as many of the animals we sought to eat or avoid. Once humans developed the mental and verbal skills to speculate about life, people found new reasons to be anxious: *Will the herds return? Will there be enough rain to keep the nut trees from dying? What will happen when I'm too old to hunt? Will my children survive after me?*

Today we live in an anxiety-ridden culture, constantly subjected to real or created bad news. The bad news also takes the form of things that haven't yet happened, including warnings and predictions about the weather, earthquakes, changes to the ozone layer, and so much more. All these things ramp up our anxiety, producing vast amounts of damaging cytokines that dramatically ratchet up the inflammatory load.

You should enlist health practitioners to provide recommendations for relaxation exercises, meditation, yoga, massage, etc. If your anxiety does not respond to these interventions, or if you find yourself turning to self-medication or other unhealthy ways of coping, see a health professional for an individual evaluation. Individual therapy or prescribed medications by a psychiatrist may be a necessary next step to jump-start the healing process.

Tools for Every Need

Look upon each modulator as a tool. Perhaps you'll need to use two or three such tools on a daily basis to maintain a positive homeostasis. But when dealing with a significant stressor, such as major illness, surgery, or psychosocial distress, you might need to add to your toolbox. Each modulator will help to some extent, but when used together, they lead to significant improvement. They all influence the way in which stress, homeostatic imbalance, and inflammation affects your body. Now we'll take a closer look at the importance of vitamers for inflammation control.

---

[72] Sheridan, J.F., Dobbs, C., Brown, D., Zwilling B., "Psychoneuroimmunology: Stress Effects on Pathogenesis and Immunity During Infection, *Clin Microbiol Rev.*, 1994; 7(2):200–212. Pitsavos, C., Anxiety in Relation to Inflammation and Coagulation Markers, among Healthy Adults: *The ATTICA Study*, 2006; 185(2):320–326.

NINE

MODULATING THE
INFLAMMATORY RESPONSE

↓Vitamers→↓Acute Inflammatory Response
↓Vitamers→↑Chronic Inflammatory Response

We've seen how inflammation plays a crucial role in health, firing up and then cooling off in response to the body's needs. When the body is in homeostatic balance, the inflammatory response works like the flame atop a brand-new gas stove, roaring to a fever pitch at a moment's notice and disappearing just as quickly. When all is well, your inflammatory response remains in the "sweet spot," flaring up to squelch infections but never becoming either the excessive inflammation leading rapidly to severe distress or the chronic inflammation killing you over the long run by triggering illnesses.

If a fine-tuned inflammation response is required to keep the body healthy, what is required to keep the inflammatory response beneficial? We talked about many factors in the previous chapter, but ample supplies of the vitamers B12 and folate are absolutely necessary as modulators of all other modulators for optimal "inflammation health." The anti-intuitive fact about a vitamer deficiency is that it can cause *both* inflammatory extremes, making the inflammatory response either wildly over-responsive or seriously under-responsive. In other words, a vitamer deficiency knocks you out of the healthy inflammatory zone in one direction or the other.

Inflamed Women, Less Inflamed Men

Before examining how a vitamer deficiency provides both an increased and a decreased inflammatory response, it's important to note that all inflammatory responses are mediated through genetics. Gender is one basic component of genetics. Women's physiology tends to have "hotter" responses while men tend to be "cooler," for good and ill. A study in the *American Journal of Pathology* notes: "Women are known to respond to infection, vaccination, and trauma with increased antibody production . . ."[73] As mentioned before, women, with their two X chromosomes, tend to have a stronger immune response. This "hotter," intensified response produces more frequent and severe bouts of inflammation and is more likely to develop into autoimmune disorders. Men, with their "cooler," one X immune reaction, tend to have a lower inflammatory response, which makes them less likely to have autoimmune illnesses but more likely to suffer from infections because their bodies don't fight pathogens as aggressively.

Being Your Own Worst Enemy

An autoimmune illness is basically the body's inability to accept its own cells, causing a full-blown immune reaction against itself. Examples of autoimmune disorders include rheumatoid arthritis, lupus erythematosus, inflammatory bowel disease, type 1 diabetes, psoriasis, and many others.

Low Vitamers in Voluntary and Involuntary Vegans

Analyzing the inflammation-related effects of an outright B12 deficiency is difficult, due to the challenge of finding a large group of people with a clear-cut, serious shortfall. With subclinical deficiencies, your various bodily systems will limp along, never presenting as symptoms severe enough to bring you in for a checkup.

There are some populations, however, who voluntarily limit their intake of B12 by declining to eat meat. Examining these groups gives us an indication of what happens with a shortage, while hinting at more subtle deficiency symptoms in the rest of us.

Studies have shown that adults maintaining a strict vegan diet suffer from a greater incidence of inflammatory illnesses. An interesting 2014 analysis looking at adult vegans found that they "are less healthy (in terms of cancer,

---

[73] Rose, N., et al, "Sex Differences in Autoimmune Disease from a Pathological Perspective," *American Journal of Pathology*, September 2008; 173(3):600–609. doi:10.2353/ajpath.2008.071008.

allergies, and mental health disorders), have a lower quality of life, and also require more medical treatment."[74] While this paper doesn't mention B12 and folate specifically, we can extrapolate that B12 would be low or absent, for it only comes from meat and seafood. It seems that whatever supplemental B12/F vegans are taking is not meeting their health needs. Deficits can show up in just four weeks on a vegan diet with reduced B12 measured.[75]

Studies have also shown that babies born to mothers who strictly adhere to veganism are at risk for a wide variety of neurodevelopmental problems.[76] The greatest risk these babies face is death from infection because their poorly functioning immune response leaves them unable to fight off these illnesses. This horrible situation has been described in child neglect cases reported in the medical literature and in the media. A tragic case occurred in France in 2008, when two strict vegans were charged in the death of their infant daughter when she developed life-threatening deficiencies of vitamins B12 and A after being fed exclusively on mother's milk.[77] The infant's poor health status was noted at her nine-month checkup, with doctors recommending that she be hospitalized for weight loss and bronchitis—her weakened system could not handle this infection. Her parents ignored the advice, did not remedy the nutrient deficiency, and their child died.

The point of all this is not to dump on vegans and vegetarians. I want to help them maximize the potential benefits of their low animal protein diets by suggesting they supplement with vitamers. I would like to see long-term health studies comparing vitamer-taking vegans and vegetarians to red meat eaters. My bet is that the vegan diet supplemented would surpass most others for promoting physical and emotional health and longevity.

Involuntary vegans are those individuals who rarely if ever eat meat because they cannot afford the cost of enough more-expensive protein with enough vitamers in it. Those forced into restricted living circumstances—prisons,

---

[74] Burkert, N.T., Muckenhuber, J., Großschädl, F., et al, "Nutrition and Health—The Association Between Eating Behavior and Various Health Parameters: A Matched Sample Study," *PLoS ONE* 9(2): e88278. doi:10.1371/journal.pone.0088278.

[75] Lederer, A., et al, "Vitamin B12 Status Upon Short-Term Intervention with a Vegan Diet—A Randomized Controlled Trial in Healthy Participants, *Nutrients*, 2019; 11(11).

[76] Di Genova, T., Harvey, G., "Infants and Children Consuming Atypical Diets: Vegetarianism and Macrobiotics, *Paediatric Child Health*, 2007, 12(3):185–188.

[77] Wilsher, Kim. "French Vegans Face Trial after Death of Baby Fed Only on Breast Milk," *The Guardian*, March 29, 2011. Accessible at http://www.theguardian.com/world/2011/mar/29/vegans-trial-death-baby-breast-milk. Viewed October 14, 2015.

nursing homes, long-term care—not supplied adequate nutrients can also be involuntary vegans.

Not-So-Intensive Care

Another population suffering the effects of low vitamers consists of patients in intensive-care units. Already under tremendous physical and psychological stress due to their illnesses, they are not being served B12/folate-rich meat and are not being given oral or injectable vitamers. However, they are getting multiple medications that stress their livers, preventing the conversion of the vitamins they do receive into vitamers. When B12 is added to the treatment regimen in critical care patients, they tend to get better quicker.[78] As the study authors noted:

> Current evidence suggests that high-dose parenteral [intravenous (IV) infusion or injection] vitamin B12 may prove an innovative approach to treat critically ill systemic inflammatory response syndrome patients, especially those with severe sepsis/septic shock [think COVID progression]. In this setting, vitamin B12 and transcobalamins [transporter proteins for B12] could modulate systemic inflammation contributing to the anti-inflammatory cascade and potentially improve outcome.

Vaccine Smokescreen

There's yet another group of people who tend to have lower B12 levels—seniors. They suffer from an age-related decrease in the ability to absorb B12, the use of multiple medications, poor supplement utilization, and chronic low-level inflammation. A fascinating study has shown how low levels of B12 and the resulting weak immune reaction suppresses the antibody response to vaccinations.

Vaccinations are designed to trigger a response from the immune system, to fool it into thinking the body is under attack and rush to develop the appropriate antibodies. Because older people are more susceptible to pneumonia caused

---

[78] Manzanares, W., Hardy, G., "Vitamin B12: The Forgotten Micronutrient for Critical Care, *Curr Opin Clin Nutr Metab Care*, 2010; 13(6):662–8.

by pneumococcal bacteria, they are given vaccinations to protect them. If the seniors have low vitamer levels, their immune response is weak, and they cannot manufacture enough antibodies in reaction to the vaccine.[79]

In essence, the vaccine is not as useful as doctor and patient believe, and the bacteria then strike with deadly force. Since vitamin levels are not regularly checked and B12 and folate are not routinely given prophylactically, many unfortunate seniors die of the very pneumonia they were supposed to be protected against. The loss in lives and healthcare funds is enormous and could be prevented with just a few dollars' worth of preventative B12 and folate.

Low Vitamers and Excessive Inflammation

The weakened inflammation response triggered by a lack of vitamers is a significant problem, matched only by the exaggerated inflammatory response caused by the same deficit. A lack of B12 and folate can cause your inflammatory response to run overly "hot," manifesting as a chronic immune response, an ongoing inflammatory battle against enemies not there.

Studies have shown that the body responds to low folate levels by manufacturing pro-inflammatory chemicals and cells. This leads to, among other things, an increased inflammatory response in the vessels of the heart and brain, causing a buildup of plaque on the inner walls of the arteries and setting the stage for heart attacks and strokes.[80] We are just now beginning to acknowledge coronary artery disease as an inflammatory process successfully modulated with B12/F and that a high blood homocysteine level, all by itself, causes an increase in the damage to the vessel walls.[81] Research has found that the body's reaction to severe infection is to produce extra B12 transporter proteins. This response evolved over millions of years so all available dietary B12 can be captured and transported into cells in preparation for repair and new cell growth. The following quote is from a journal article written by Dr. Carmen Wheatley in which she suggests that:

> [Vitamin B12] . . . is central to the effectiveness of the immune
> inflammatory response and that its deficiency, chronic, functional or

---

[79] Fata, F.T., Herzlich, B.C., Schiffman, G., Ast, A.L., "Impaired Antibody Responses to Pneumococcal Polysaccharide in Elderly Patients with Low Serum Vitamin B12 Levels," *Annals of Internal Medicine*, 1996; 124(3):229–304.

[80] Kolb, A.F., Peitrie L., "Folate Deficiency Enhances the Inflammatory Response of Macrophages," *Mol Immunol*, 2013; 54(2):164–72.

[81] Moat, S.J., Sagar N., Doshi, D.L., et al, "Treatment of Coronary Heart Disease with Folic Acid: Is There a Future?" *American Journal of Physiology—Heart and Circulatory Physiology*, 2004; 287(1):H1–H7.

"compartmental," may largely contribute to the etiology [cause] of systemic inflammatory response system (SIRS)/sepsis/septic shock, as well as autoimmune disease, central nervous system (CNS) disease, cancer, in particular haematological malignancy, and the progression of AIDS.[82]

The concept of using folate to reduce inflammation was tested in a study of sixty healthy but overweight volunteers. Remember, excess adipose tissue uses a lot of extra folate. Those who were given folate enjoyed a reduction in the levels of certain inflammatory mediators, despite the fact that they did not significantly reduce their fat mass/BMI. The results of this study (with the less efficient folic acid) suggest a role for folate in reducing the inflammation that sets the stage for heart disease and strokes.[83]

Now that we've seen how a lack of vitamers cause inflammation to run either too "hot" or too "cool," let's focus in on how these might influence the course of three major health concerns: cancer, mental health, and pain.

Vitamers, Inflammation, and Cancer

Many forms of cancer begin as an inflammatory process. My grandfather died of esophageal cancer, even though he did not indulge in either of the two main causes of throat cancer—smoking or consuming alcohol. He did, however, drink boiling hot espresso coffee every day of his adult life. This repeated application of scalding water to a sensitive body tissue is a pro-inflammatory risk factor leading to the formation of cancer and his eventual death.

In an article titled "Inflammation and Cancer," two researchers point out:

Recent data have expanded the concept that inflammation is a critical component of tumour progression. Many cancers arise from sites of infection, chronic irritation and inflammation. It is now becoming clear

---

[82] See, for example, 1) Wheatley, C., "A Scarlet Pimpernel for the Resolution Of Inflammation? The Role of Supra-Therapeutic Doses of Cobalamin, in the Treatment of Systemic Inflammatory Response Syndrome (SIRS), Sepsis, Severe Sepsis, and Septic or Traumatic Shock," *Medical Hypotheses*, 2006; 67(1):124–42, and 2) Wheatley, C., "The Return of the Scarlet Pimpernel: Cobalamin in Inflammation II: Cobalamins Can Both Selectively Promote All Three Nitric Oxide Synthases (NOS), Particularly iNOS and eNOS, and, as Needed, Selectively Inhibit iNOS and nNOS," *J Nutr Environ Med*, 2007;1 6(3–4):181–211.

[83] Solini, A., Santini, E., Ferrannini, E., "Effect of Short-Term Folic Acid Supplementation on Insulin Sensitivity and Inflammatory Markers in Overweight Subjects," *Int J Obes (Lond)*, 2006; (8):1197–202.

that the tumour microenvironment, which is largely orchestrated by inflammatory cells, is an indispensable participant in the neoplastic [new cancer cell growth] process, fostering proliferation, survival and migration.[84]

This is not new news. Back in the 1850s, Germany's Dr. Rudolf Virchow, who established the study of cellular pathology, noted that disease involves alterations in normal cells and that cancer is closely associated with the presence of an inflammatory process.[85] His studies led to later observations that chronic inflammation from any cause, including obesity, infection, or toxins, increases the threat of cancer development. Further observations indicated that inflammation "encourages" cancer at each stage of its development. Actively reducing inflammation—at any stage in the cancer process—prompts better outcomes.

An article in the *British Medical Journal* neatly sums up the situation and points out that reducing inflammation may be a powerful weapon against cancer:

> [T]he conditions provided by a chronic inflammatory environment are so essential for the progression of the neoplastic process that therapeutic intervention aimed at inhibiting inflammation, reducing angiogenesis [growth of new blood vessels in developing tumors] and stimulating cell mediated immune responses may have a major role in reducing the incidence of common cancers.[86]

Having ample supplies of B12 and folate helps reduce cancer-causing inflammation. In addition, these two nutrients play an essential role in DNA formation, reducing the damage caused by toxins we are exposed to in the food we eat and the air we breathe. Ensuring that DNA is properly formed can help guard against certain cancers. A great many studies show that low levels of B12 and folate are linked to various forms of cancer. For example:

- *Colorectal cancer* – The famous Nurses' Health Study, which was begun in 1976, has followed over 120,000 nurses for many years.

---

[84] Coussens, L.M., Werb, Z., "Inflammation and Cancer," *Nature*, 2002; 420:860–867.
[85] Grivennikov, S.I., Freten, F.R., Karin, M., et al, "Immunity, Inflammation, and Cancer," *Cell*, 2010; 140(6):883–899.
[86] O'Byrne, K.J., Dalgleish. A.G., "Chronic Immune Activation And Inflammation as the Cause of Malignancy," *Br J Cancer*, 2001;85(4):473–483.

Researchers discovered an increased risk of colon cancer in those deficient in folate and that a "high intake of folate may reduce risk for colon cancer."[87]

- *Breast cancer* – A study of postmenopausal women found that a "high folate intake was associated with decreased breast cancer risk. Vitamin B12 intake may modify this association."[88] In another study, folic acid and vitamin B12 were found to be protective against *BRCA*-associated breast cancer.[89] (If folic acid worked well in this study, how much better would folate work?)

- *Lung cancer* – A study comparing 470 people with lung cancer to control patients who did not have the cancer found that consuming foods rich in folate led to a 40 percent reduction in the risk of developing the disease.[90] The risk of developing cancer was greater in those with low folate who also consumed alcohol on a regular basis. This is no surprise, for alcohol and cigarettes are known to be synergistic pro-inflammatory factors, in which one factor plus another factor has the ill effect equal to three factors.

- *Esophageal, gastric, and pancreatic cancer* – A meta-analysis (study of studies) combined the results of multiple findings to create a single, larger, and more powerful look at a disease. It found that compromised levels of folate in the blood, whether due to inadequate intake or reduced MTHFR-enzyme activity, significantly increases the risk of developing a variety of intestinal system cancers.[91] The lower the level of folate, the greater the risk of these abnormal growths.

- *Cervical cancer* – Studies have found an inverse relationship between serum folate and B12 levels on the one hand, and the incidence of

[87] Giovannucci, E, et al, "Multivitamin Use, Folate, and Colon Cancer in Women in the Nurses' Health Study," *Annals of Internal Medicine*, October 1, 1998; 129(7):517–24.

[88] Lajous, M., et al, Folate, Vitamin B12 and Postmenopausal Breast Cancer in a Prospective Study of French Women," *Cancer Causes Control*, 2006; 17(9):1209–13.

[89] Kim, S.J., et al, "Folic Acid Supplement Use and Breast Cancer Risk in BRCA1 and BRCA2 Mutation Carriers: A Case-Control Study," *Breast Cancer Res Treat*, April 2019;174(3):741–748.

[90] Shen, H., et al, "Dietary Folate Intake and Lung Cancer Risk in Former Smokers: A Case-Control Analysis," Cancer Epidemiol Biomarkers Prev, 2003; 12(10):980–6.

[91] Larsson, S.C., Giovannucci, E., Wolk, A., "Folate Intake, MTHFR Polymorphisms, and Risk of Esophageal, Gastric, and Pancreatic Cancer: A Meta-Analysis," *Gastroenterology*, 2006; 131(4):1271–1283.

abnormal cells of the cervix and the development of cervical cancer on the other.[92, 93] Ironically, in addition to a greater risk of malignancy with low B12/F, there is also an increased risk of false positive pre-cancer reports (dysplasia) found in cervical cell sampling (PAP smears). In other words, the vitamer deficiency that makes cervical cells more at risk for conversion to cancer also makes the cells look precancerous when they are not.[94]

Additional MTHFR Risk

An additional risk for developing any kind of cancer comes from the genetic mutation causing decreased MTHFR function, preventing the conversion of folic acid into folate and creating low serum folate.[95]

Stealth Mental Health

A lack of B12 and folate does more than harm your physical health. Vitamer deficiency triggers damage to your nervous system, contributing to cognitive disturbance (dementia) and emotional health symptoms such as depression and anxiety. These most often appear long before the vitamer-deficient anemia shows up as abnormal on a test. These deficiencies are stealthy ways mental health is worsened over time and rarely identified or treated.

Inflammation may harm brain function on two levels.[96] First, it reduces the electrical communication between nerve connections by hindering the function of the myelin sheaths protecting the nerves. Second, it reduces biochemical communication by elevating the level of pro-inflammatory proteins such as cytokines while reducing neurotransmitter production. Patients with anxiety, mania, and depression have been found to have

---

[92] Tong, S., Kim, M.K., Lee, J.W., et al, "Common Polymorphisms in Methylenetetrahydrofolate Reductase Gene Are Associated with Risks of Cervical Intraepithelial Neoplasia and Cervical Cancer in Women with Low Serum Folate and Vitamin B12," *Cancer Causes & Control*, 2011; 22(1):63–72.

[93] Butterworth, C.E. Jr., et al, "Folate Deficiency and Cervical Dysplasia," *JAMA*, January 22–29,1992; 267(4):528–33.

[94] Yüksel, H., et al, "Folate and Vitamin B12 Levels in Abnormal Pap Smears: A Case Control Study, *Eur J Gynaecol Oncol*, 2007; 28(6):526–30.

[95] Lei-Zhou Xia, et al, "Methylenetetrahydrofolate Reductase C677T and A1298C Polymorphisms and Gastric Cancer Susceptibility," *World Journal of Gastroenterology*, August 28, 2014; 20(32): 11429–11438.

[96] Raison, C.L., Capuron, L., Miller, A.H., "Cytokines Sing the Blues: Inflammation and the Pathogenesis of Depression," *Trends Immunol*, 2006; 27(1):24–31.

significantly higher levels of these cytokines. These proteins interfere with neurotransmitters and neuroendocrine communication, leading to various mental health and dementia challenges.

Mania is just one of these challenges. In one case-report, an eighty-one-year-old man with a B12 deficiency had what appeared to be mania, yet he responded to vitamin B12 supplements without the need for long-term psychiatric medication or a recurrence of his illness.[97] In another case, a thirty-five-year-old woman developed the classic symptoms of mania and was admitted for evaluation and treatment. Her lab tests were within normal limits except for a significantly low blood B12 level, and her physical exam was normal except for some minor neurologic abnormalities. The doctors thought she had a seizure disorder and treated her accordingly, with little benefit. When her low B12 was finally diagnosed and treated, her manic episodes disappeared in three days, and her abnormal neurologic signs vanished in a month.[98]

These are not isolated cases, for low levels of vitamers have been linked to mood disorders in a number of studies. Among these disorders is depression, with an unknown number of sufferers who may be relieved of their distress with a simple improvement in vitamin intake. Indeed, one of the most common symptoms of B12/folate deficiency is depression, because the vitamers are essential to the manufacture of SAMe (S-adenosylmethionine), which makes the chemical messengers, the neurotransmitters regulating mood.

All of the following neurotransmitters listed on the graphic below are B12 and folate dependent.

NEUROTRANSMITTERS

ADRENALINE	GABA
fight or flight	calming
produced in stressful situations. Increases heart rate and blood flow, leading to physical boost and heightened awareness.	Calms firing nerves in the central nervous system. High levels improve focus, low levels cause anxiety. Also contributes to motor control and vision.
NORADRENALINE	ACETYLCHOLINE
concentration	learning
affects attention and responding actions in the brain. Contracts blood vessels, increasing blood flow.	Involved in thought, learning and memory. Activates muscle action in the body. Also associated with attention and awakening.
DOPAMINE	GLUTAMATE
pleasure	memory
feelings of pleasure, also addiction, movement and motivation. People repeat behaviors that lead to dopamine release.	Most common neurotransmitter. Involved in learning and memory, regulates development and creation of nerve contacts.
SEROTONIN	ENDORPHINS
mood	euphoria
contributes to well-being and happiness. Helps sleep cycle and digestive system regulation. Affected by exercise and light exposure.	Released during exercise, excitement and sex, producing well-being and euphoria, reducing pain

---

[97] Goggans, F. C., "A Case of Mania Secondary to Vitamin B_{12} Deficiency," *American Journal of Psychiatry*, 1984; 141(2):300–301.

[98] Gomez-Bernal, G. J., Milagros Bernal-Perez, M., "Vitamin B12 Deficiency Manifested as Mania: A Case Report," *Journal of Clinical Psychiatry*, 2007; 9(3):238.

In essence, B12/F deficiency worsens mental health and neurologic problems in five ways:

- Myelin production decreases, and the nerve cells communicate inefficiently.

- Homocysteine increases, increasing inflammation in the brain.

- MAO released from the immature platelets of deficiency shortens the life of neurotransmitters so messages between brain cells are slowed.

- DNA-methylation is reduced so there is a reduction in the coordinated expression of the genes, leading to poor functioning and aging of the brain cells.

- Neurotransmitter production decreases because the precursor SAMe can't be made.

There are reports of a reduced incidence of depression in populations consuming a high-folate diet. More interesting, the response to the treatment of depression with antidepressants is muted in populations low in vitamers. Connecting the dots created by numerous findings such as these makes it clear that B12 and folate are absolutely necessary for good mental health. Indeed, a review of a wide variety of patients has shown B12 and/or folate deficiency results in a significant increase in depressive symptoms, and treatment with these agents leads to better outcomes.[99]

In addition to psychiatric symptoms, long-term inflammatory processes triggered by deficiency lead to cognitive decline. In a review article appearing in the *British Medical Journal*,[100] Dr. Reynolds pointed out that:

- Folate helps regulate cognition, mood, and social function.

- A lack of folate is linked to depression and dementia.

- Difficulty metabolizing folate may trigger "a pattern of cognitive dysfunction that resembles ageing."

- Among the elderly, a "deficiency contributes to ageing brain processes, increases the risk of Alzheimer's disease and vascular dementia and, if critically severe, can lead to an irreversible dementia."

[99] Coppen, A, Bolander-Gouaille, C., "Treatment of Depression: Time to Consider Folic Acid and Vitamin B12," *Journal of Psychopharmacology* 2005; 19(1):59–65.
[100] Reynolds, E.H., "Folic Acid, Ageing, Depression, and Dementia," *British Medical Journal*, 2002; 324(7352):1512–1515.

Hold the MAO

The type of anemia caused by a B12/folate deficiency, megaloblastic anemia, causes the production of too many immature platelets, which in turn spew out excess amounts of an enzyme called monoamine oxidase (MAO). This enzyme, it so happens, also speeds the breakdown of neurotransmitters in the synapses between nerve cells. This means that a B12/folate deficiency inhibits neurotransmitter levels in two significant ways: by limiting the production of SAMe, the precursor to the neurotransmitters serotonin, dopamine, and norepinephrine, and by increasing the production of MAO, which hastens their breakdown.

Elevated blood levels of the MAO enzyme have been found in those suffering from depression, postpartum depression, Parkinson's disease, Alzheimer's disease, and bipolar disorder. It makes sense that if you could block this enzyme in the chemical junction between nerves called synapses, you would have higher level of neurotransmitters and maybe less depression. And that is exactly what researchers developed—MAO inhibitors as antidepressants were one of the first pharmaceutical approaches used to treat depression.

Pain Reduction

The human body is awash in small proteins called cytokines that play a key role in the immune system's response to danger. Although these cytokines are necessary for good health, they have their potential downside. Scientific evidence indicates that they initiate and/or prolong pain by activating nerve cells designed to detect and respond to painful stimuli. Certain cytokines also play a role in triggering a chronic painful condition called *central sensitization*, in which pain exists for no apparent physical reason.[101] B12 and folate, with their anti-inflammatory actions, work directly on moderating this kind of inflammatory response and reduce any persistent pain related to inflammation.[102]

---

[101] Zhang, J.M., An, J., "Cytokines, Inflammation and Pain," *Int. Anesthesiol Clin*, 2007; 45(2):27–37.
[102] Mikkelsen, Kathleen, et al, "Vitamin B12, Folic Acid, and the Immune System," *Nutrition and Immunity*, July 31, 2019, 103–114.

Animal studies have shown that B12 is an effective anti-inflammatory and anti-pain agent, and research confirms this is also true in humans.[103] For example:

- Italian researchers evaluated B12's ability to reduce back pain in sixty adults suffering from inflammation of the sciatic nerve called *sciatic neuritis*.[104] They found that injections of B12 reduced the amount of pain medication the volunteers required to function better.

- In a study published in 1994, researchers worked with twenty-six individuals suffering from osteoarthritis to see if reducing their joint inflammation with B12 and folate would lessen their pain.[105] One-third of the volunteers were given B12 and folate, another one-third received NSAIDS, and the remaining one-third took a placebo. Repeated testing of hand-grip strength showed that those taking the two vitamers enjoyed just as much benefit as those taking the NSAIDs. However, there was an advantage to using the nutrients, which was a greater reduction in the number of painful joints. In addition, the vitamers triggered no side effects, while the NSAIDs were responsible for many unfortunate consequences.

- The effects of B12 were tested on one hundred people suffering from diabetic neuropathy, which arises from damage to the nerve connections triggered by diabetes.[106] This can cause crippling pain, plus the feeling of electrical shocks and burning sensations not helped by most standard treatments. For this study, B12 was compared to a standard pain-reducing agent and antidepressant called nortriptyline. The fifty volunteers receiving the B12 enjoyed a fourfold (400 percent) greater reduction in pain perception than did those taking the standard medicine. It's interesting to note that one of the popular medicines for type 2 diabetes, metformin, suppresses B12 levels,

---

[103] Hosseinzadeh H, et al, "Anti-Nociceptive and Anti-Inflammatory Effects of Cyanocobalamin (Vitamin B12) Against Acute and Chronic Pain and Inflammation in Mice," *Arzneimittelforschung*, 2012; 62(7):324–9.

[104] Mauro, G.L., et al, "Vitamin B12 in Low Back Pain: A Randomised, Double-Blind, Placebo-Controlled Study," *Eur Rev Med Pharmacol Sci*, 2000; 4(3):53–8.

[105] Flynn, M.A., Irvin, W., Krause, G., "The Effect of Folate and Cobalamin on Osteoarthritis Hands," *J Am Coll Nutr*, 1994; 13(4):351–356.

[106] Talaei, A., Siavash, M., Majidi, H., Cherhrei, A., "Vitamin B12 May Be More Effective Than Nortriptyline in Improving Painful Diabetic Neuropathy," *Int J Food Sci Nutr*, 2009; 60(Suppl 5):71–76.

thereby increasing the nerve pain from diabetic neuropathy.[107] This indicates that this popular treatment for type 2 diabetes is really a hidden cause of worsening the pain of peripheral neuropathy.

There are many other studies showing that B12 and folate help reduce pain. Their ability to do so is all the more important when you consider the Food and Drug Administration's July 2015 statement that even low doses of the NSAIDs used for pain can make some people more susceptible to strokes and heart attacks. These are serious, often fatal problems. Since B12 and folate reduce pain in many people suffering from a variety of painful ailments, shouldn't they be offered as an alternative or adjunct to pain medicines?

Pain Reframe

Just understanding the following will allow you to reframe and reduce the severity of intermittent or chronic pain experiences for the rest of your life. Pain is merely a message to the brain to pay attention, an alert that something is not right. Once this message is received, the brain tells the whole body to do something, anything, to reduce the likelihood of continued pain and injury: "That stove is hot, so move your hand now or there will be permanent damage." The signal to and from the brain itself does not cause any physical damage, though it "feels" like it does.

There are different sources of pain, and adults and children should be educated about these. If the pain message is from a broken wrist that has been set and fit with a cast, then any pain signals to and from the brain that continue are redundant. You have done and are doing everything to care for the source of pain, and there is nothing else to do, so further signals can be ignored as much as possible. No new information is coming from the brain—a reinterpretation of the signal is necessary.

Then there is another kind of pain—the "helping pain" of shots, physical therapy, etc. When I would give shots to children, their anxious parent would say as I was standing there with a needle: "This won't hurt." I immediately corrected them in front of their child, saying, "This will hurt. You can yell and cry all you want, but it is a helping hurt, and if you hold very still, we can get it over with very quick."

---

[107] Bell, D.S., "Metformin-Induced Vitamin B12 Deficiency Presenting as a Peripheral Neuropathy," *South Med J*, 2010; 103(3):265–267.

A Role for Vitamers in HIV/AIDS?

If low vitamer levels cause your immune response to run "cold," you are more susceptible to infections because you cannot make enough antibodies and killer white blood cells to fight off invaders. This means that an unknown number of patients with AIDS (Acquired Immune Deficiency Syndrome) have the double challenge of immune deficiency caused by HIVplus the vitamer deficiency triggered by the medications used in treatment.

In these affected patients, the problem is not just a vulnerability to a wide variety of infections; it is also the fact the infections develop more quickly in those who are vitamer-deficient. According to a Johns Hopkins University research study, low levels of these vitamers allow an HIV infection to progress to AIDS four years sooner than those with normal vitamer intake.[108] While this does not suggest that B12 can prevent AIDS, it should be of interest to treating professionals and those who have the disease. Simply staving off the progression for several years can produce tremendous benefits, for a modest investment.

Pulling It All Together

In this chapter we reviewed the role of the B vitamers in maintaining homeostatic balance and the importance of keeping the inflammatory response in the "sweet spot," neither too "hot" nor too "cold." We reviewed some of the illnesses associated with low vitamers in the blood and treatment with vitamers to reduce medical problems. In the next chapter, we'll look at the few basic dietary means of controlling excessive inflammation.

---

[108] Tang, A.M., Graham, N.M., Chandra, R.K., Saah, A.J., "Low Serum Vitamin B-12 Concentrations Are Associated with Faster Human Immunodeficiency Virus Type 1 (HIV-1) Disease Progression," *Journal of Nutrition*, 1997; 129(2):345–351.

TEN

TAMING THE BEAST WITHIN—
DIETARY MODULATORS

↑Adipose Tissue →↑ WBC, ↑Cytokines, ↓Vitamers→
↑Chronic Inflammation →↓Health

Most of us can afford to lose some weight, but more importantly, we all have a need to shed some inflammation. Adipose (fat) cells are inflammation-generating tissues in the body. We need to reduce foods that add to the inflammation caused by adipose (fat) tissue while simultaneously getting more foods that are anti-inflammatory. I recommend that you start a food fight against inflammation by using food to reduce your inflammatory load. Doing so will improve your health immediately and over the long run. Rather than thinking about pounds, keep your focus on your health, on feeling better, and on living longer. Think of eating and taking inflammatory-reducing vitamers as part of a larger health plan, letting the pounds fall as they may.

Adipose Cells, Inflammation, and Vitamers

Excess adipose tissue reduces serum folate levels and triggers the excess production of cytokines and pro-inflammatory molecules throughout every body organ and tissue. At some point, varying from person to person, fat cells take on a gluttonous life of their own. They demand glucose, prompting those late-night trips to get carbohydrate/sugar treats. For some folks, their bodies' demand for more and more glucose become so powerful and incessant they take precedence over work, relationships, self-esteem, and health, making them eat when and what they don't need to. And of course, the more calories consumed, the larger and more controlling the beast grows.

There are three primary places where excess adipose cells congregate: in the abdomen beneath the abdominal muscles, between muscle and liver tissue cells, and under the skin. The most pro-inflammatory fat is the kind packed into the abdomen, the "visceral fat" surrounding internal organs. This surplus adipose tissue is a veritable inflammation-production machine. B12 and folate deficiencies encourage the buildup of fat in this deadly area. This is a feedback loop affecting fat deposition on an epigenetic level, encouraging obesity, the development of insulin resistance, diabetes, and, naturally, more inflammation.

Fat cells are the second most abundant tissue in the body behind skeletal muscle in most individuals. These cells can become the most predominant tissue in the body of some, putting them into a more unhealthy, pro-inflammatory homeostasis.

There are three kinds of fat cells: white, brown, and an intermediate form called beige. The main difference is the number of mitochondria present in each cell. If there is one, the cell is white; when there are a few mitochondria, the cells look beige; and when there are many, the cell is called brown. The more mitochondria a cell has, the more energy it produces. The other main difference is that the white cells are 99 percent of the adipose cells in an adult, with brown and beige making up the difference. While great at storage, the white fat cells do little to turn stored energy into heat. Brown fat cells are expert at this, putting out significant heat energy. Evolution has made them so efficient; they are found in high numbers in newborns to create enough heat to survive childbirth and the perilous postnatal period. By the time adulthood has arrived, the cells have died out except for a small patch between the shoulder blades. A beige fat cell is an intermediate kind that has some storage properties and some heat-producing properties. Individuals with more active brown and beige cells have a greater resistance to obesity and diabetes, with some of these having constitutional thinness. These individuals have mitochondria in their adipose cells that are very active, making more energy burning up the fat.[109] Imagine how well the mitochondria of your adipose cells would burn fat if they had all the B vitamers they needed!

Reducing a major source of inflammation—adipose tissue—should be a key objective of any eating plan. This is especially important for those hoping

---

[109] Ling, Y., et al., "Persistent low Body Weight In Humans Is Associated with Higher Mitochondrial Activity in White Adipose Tissue," *American Journal of Clinical Nutrition*, 2019; 110:605–616.

to have children.[110] Men and women who are overweight at the time of conception will have an increased inflammatory load, putting their offspring at greater risk of developing early death from all causes later in their life.[111] Adipose tissue is a major source of inflammation and an actual endocrine organ because it produces so many pro-inflammatory proteins (cytokines, leptin, sex steroids), which leads to insulin resistance.

"The Four Ws" of Anti-Inflammatory Weight Control

In a country of plenty, food consumption is often driven more by emotions than by hunger. Family, culture, fashion, and stress all inform what and how we eat. The complexity of the topic is beyond the scope of this book other than clarifying the importance of learning how to eat for long-term needs of the body rather than for short-term emotions.

Instead of the never-ending quest to find "the best diet," I suggest you focus on the Four Ws of eating: Why, When, What, and Where. Once understood and integrated into a daily routine, you will create an eating regimen that's uniquely anti-inflammatory for you.

The "Why" of Eating

If you are in reasonable health, there is only one good reason to eat, and that is because you are hungry. It sounds obvious, but most of us eat for all kinds of reasons having little to do with the body's requirement for nutrition. Because "it's time," someone else is eating, we're anxious, the food is free, or if we don't eat it, it will only go to waste are all typical examples.

When the opportunity to eat arises, make an effort to ask yourself this simple question: "Am I hungry?"

Most of us have forgotten what it's like to feel true hunger. Anxiety about getting enough food to survive another day has been a part of all animal evolution since the beginning of animals. Evolution has primed us to feel anxious when we're in need of food, so we'll go searching for something to eat. This anxiety is such a part of us that we all unconsciously associate any source of anxiety with the need for nourishment.

Today, most of us in the developed countries know where our next meal

---

[110] Pasquali, R., "Obesity, Fat Distribution and Infertility," *Maturitas*, Volume 54, Issue 4, 20 July 2006, 363–371.
[111] McPherson, N., "Peri-Conception Parental Obesity, Reproductive Health, and Transgenerational Impacts," *Trends in Endocrinology & Metabolism*, Volume 26, Issue 2, February 2015, 84–90.

is coming from, making food anxiety unnecessary, but we still do our best to avoid even a twinge of hunger-anxiety. Instead of fearing the sensation, we should embrace it, using it as a tool to tell us when we really need to consume calories. Hunger is a neuro-endocrine signal like thirst or pain, but it's just that—a signal. And just like the signal of pain, the signal itself doesn't cause any damage to your body. You can choose to respond to this indicator at what you consider is an appropriate time, rather than running to the refrigerator at the first little flicker.

The "When" of Eating

How do you know when you're hungry and when you just feel like eating? Learning to recognize the difference is important. Start by making a ten-point list that spells out your different levels of hunger. Here's an example:

1- Stuffed

2- Full

3- Satiated

4- "In a little while, I'll be hungry"

5- "I could eat"

6- Peckish

7- Hungry

8- Famished

9- Ravenous

10- Starving

Come up with your own list. Keep it with you until you have learned it by heart (or by stomach) so you can instantly tune into your true hunger level. Then eat only when your hunger rises to a seven on *your* scale.

And what about the rest of the time? Is it really a good idea to wait until you're feeling hungry before you refuel? It is, for while you are in the fasting (non-eating, non-digesting) state your body doesn't have to devote energy and attention to dealing with incoming food. In other words, the body has been nourished, and the disruptions caused by digestion, assimilation, and the resulting changes in blood levels of various nutrients and other substances have been normalized. It's as if a footwear factory received a massive shipment of leather, rubber, eyelets, and other raw materials and had to spend a couple of hours storing everything in its place. Now, with everything put away, the factory can resume manufacturing shoes. Your body can get back to energy and cell production to keep everything in homeostasis.

This is a healthful state and a great time for you to *not* eat. Doing so is a distraction for your metabolic machinery. Despite the advice of those who promote consumption of six small meals at regular intervals throughout the day, the human body is not designed to process food 24/7. It needs some down time, for example, to rid itself of sick and dying cells and replace them with new ones. The body's hormone and energy cycles can focus on either exercise and building new cells or on processing just eaten food—not both efficiently.

When food is ever present, handling it takes priority over waste removal and rebuilding. Waste, like homocysteine, builds up, resulting in an increased inflammatory load. Giving the body a break from food processing allows mouth and gut bacteria, hormones, insulin levels, and nervous system time to return to a baseline homeostatic level. A constant supply of calories feeds unhealthy bacterial growth in our whole digestive tract from mouth to colon, overwhelming the healthy, less "hungry" bacteria we should try to cultivate in our intestines.

Another *when*. Science now supports the idea of a "food delay." Laboratory studies have shown eating at specific times during the day and fasting at other times (referred to as *intermittent fasting* or *time-restricted eating*) allows the body to metabolize fat more efficiently. In one study a number of mice were divided into two groups and fed the exact same number of calories. One group was given food throughout the day, while the other was restricted to food consumption during one eight-hour window. Although both consumed the same quantity of food, the group that ate throughout the day gained weight and was more susceptible to inflammatory illnesses than the time-restricted group.[112] A review of intermittent fasting in adults showed similar benefits, with improved longevity and a reduction in cancer and obesity.[113]

If, for example, you finish dinner by 7:30 p.m. and eat nothing until you break your fast with breakfast at 7:30 a.m., you are giving your body twelve hours of health-enhancing "down time." However, if you snack through the

---

[112] Hatori, M., et al, "Time-Restricted Feeding without Reducing Caloric Intake Prevents Metabolic Diseases in Mice Fed a High-Fat Diet," *Cell Metabolism*, 2012; 15(6):848–60.

[113] Cabo, R., and Mattson, M., "Effects of Intermittent Fasting on Health, Aging, and Disease," *New England Journal of Medicine*, Dec. 26, 2019; 381:2541–2551.

evening, even a little, you won't get the benefits of the fast. There is no magic number of hours required, but the longer the overnight and early morning delay, the greater the benefits.

How Time-Restricted Eating Helps You Lose Weight

After you eat dinner, the carbohydrates you've consumed are converted by the liver into glycogen, a source of quick energy to be used over the next twelve hours or so. While you sleep and for some time after you awaken, your body uses that glycogen as the primary energy source for brain and body functions. As soon as you ingest more than fifty calories worth of carbohydrates, the liver "realizes" that there is a new intake of energy, so the glycogen is no longer "needed" as an energy source and is converted into stored fat. If you delay your food intake in the morning and your body uses up its stored glycogen in the liver, it will move on to its next but less-efficient source of energy, which is previously stored fat. Using this energy source will shrink your adipose cells and will shrink your inflammatory load.

You can accelerate the fat-burning process with morning exercise, which speeds up the consumption of glycogen accumulated from your last meal the previous evening. After exercise burns up the glycogen, your body shifts to fat-burning mode until registering the intake of food energy with your next meal. If your next meal is breakfast, there won't be much time for fat-burning to occur. If it's lunch, you will have burned fat for several hours. The longer the fast between meals, the longer the fat-burning time.

Although this approach works for many people, if skipping breakfast or any other meal causes any physical distress such as heart palpitations, fatigue, anxiety, or irritability, do not delay meals and check in with your physician. Instead of delay, focus on refraining from eating anything between meals.

If I had to summarize the *when* of eating into one simple rule that works for almost anyone, it would be this: *Delay your first food ingestion and no caloric intake after 7:30 p.m.*

The "What" of Eating

One of the best presentations of basic food guidelines is offered very succinctly by Michael Pollan, author of *Food Rules: An Eater's Manual.*[114] He writes: "Eat food. Not too much. Mostly plants." In other words, you should eat real food arriving at your table fresh from the closest farm with the fewest processing steps in between. He adds a few more rules I summarize as follows: Don't overcook;

---

[114] Michael Pollan, *Food Rules: An Eater's Manual* (New York: Penguin Books, 2013).

you lose nutrients. And make vegetables, seeds, nuts, and fruits the mainstay of your diet, with smaller amounts of meat, dairy, seafood, and grains.

When you eat mostly plants, as Pollan suggests, you ensure that you get plenty of fiber. Like fish using flotsam to hide in the ocean from bigger fish, *good* bacteria use fibers to hide from *bad* bacteria that eat them and out-reproduce them. These *bad* bacteria are unhealthy because they worsen your inflammatory load.

Another way to keep blood sugar under control is to eat foods that have a low glycemic load. You may be aware of the *glycemic index*, a number assigned to a food that indicates its effect on your blood glucose—how quickly or slowly your blood sugar rises when you eat the food. Foods with high glycemic values release their sugar rapidly, while those with a low number do so slowly. Pure glucose, the standard against which everything is measured, has a value of one hundred. A baked potato is pretty high at eighty-five, popcorn at seventy, white rice at sixty-four, potato chips at fifty-four, oranges at forty-eight, apples at thirty-eight, and peanuts at fifteen. Remember, these numbers apply to the foods without added sugar, sauces, etc.

The glycemic index is an interesting approach, but even better is a measurement called the *glycemic load*, which takes into account how quickly the blood sugar rises but also how much carbohydrate is in a certain amount of food. The difference is key: not how rapidly the food releases its sugar, but what effect specific food in a specific amount will raise your blood sugar level.

The difference is not always obvious. For instance, watermelon is loaded with the sugar called fructose and has little fiber to slow its digestion, so you might think it would pump your blood sugar way up. Because watermelon is mostly composed of water, the fructose is "diluted," and one-half cup of the fruit produces a low-glycemic load of four. Carrots are another example of a sweet food with a low-glycemic load. And popcorn, with a glycemic index of seventy-two, has a glycemic load of only seven. On the other end of the scale, white rice and potato chips may not seem sweet, but they have high-glycemic loads.

Don't Get Weighed Down by Glycemic Load

The glycemic load of a food is calculated by multiplying the grams of carbohydrate in a serving of that food by its glycemic index, then divide by one hundred. For example, a cup of white rice provides fifty-two grams of carbs and has a glycemic index of sixty-four. In formula form, this is 52 x 64 = 3,328. Divide this by one hundred to come up with a glycemic load of thirty-three.

I recommend that my patients select foods with low-glycemic loads whenever possible. Rather than obsessing over food choices, just choose those with a low load over those with higher loads. The following list gives a brief idea of the wide variation of glycemic indexes and glycemic loads:

	High-Glycemic Index	High-Glycemic Load
Glucose	100	50
Baked Potato	85	28
White Rice	64	33

	High-Glycemic Index	Low-Glycemic Load
Watermelon	72	8
Popcorn	72	7

	Low-Glycemic Index	Low-Glycemic Load
Apples	38	6
Bean Sprouts	28	1
Peanuts	14	2

As for inflammation, it would be nice if we had an "inflammation index" or "inflammation load" chart to tell us which foods to embrace and which to avoid. We do know that certain foods, in general, are more pro-inflammatory (i.e., they worsen inflammation rather than cause it) or less inflammatory. Pro-inflammatory foods include white bread, white rice, pasta, processed meats, and certain food ingredients, including saturated fats, trans-fats, concentrated fructose, and some additives that encourage inflammation. Other foods, such as fatty fish, fruits, nuts, leafy vegetables, and olive oil, appear to have promising anti-inflammatory properties, but the jury is still out. You can study the various food lists to create a diet with a low-glycemic load and containing foods with possible anti-inflammatory properties, or simply follow Pollan's advice: "Eat food. Not too much. Mostly plants."

The "Where" of Eating

By "where," I don't mean in the kitchen or in the bedroom. Instead, I'm referring to where you are on your current weight curve when you begin your own inflammation/weight-control reduction. Everyone is at a different point on their own unique curve.

Imagine a graph with a curvy line representing the natural up-and-down transitions in your weight. You begin your efforts at weight reduction, and the curvy line drops down as time passes and weight is lost. You are now at a new plateau, a new steady state, a flat area of your weight-loss graph. In dietary terms, plateaus are those times when body weight stubbornly stabilizes and you're unable to lose more without making a major change.

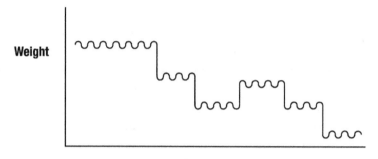

Weight

Time (weeks to months)

You may have experienced this resistance yourself while dieting. You began quickly, lost some weight, then got "stuck." The body is always trying to remain in a previous homeostasis even when the status quo is unhealthy. When you lose weight, your metabolism may slow, burning less energy to keep your weight from falling further. This makes sense from an evolutionary point of view: After all, in our distant past, holding on to body weight was very important. But evolution makes reducing inflammation/weight that much harder.

If the *where* on the curve is you at a plateau and happy with your new weight, then keep the modulators you are using to maintain that range. When you find yourself at a long plateau you don't like, don't worry—it's not your fault, you're not a failure, and most importantly, your eating regime has not failed you. This is the place on your curve where you will need to apply all the tools in your toolbox of modulators. Stay with it, make adjustments as necessary, and look forward to your next plateau breakthrough. Meanwhile, keep sleeping well, increase exercise some, and think about modestly extending your fasting periods.

For most people, it takes about five days at a new lower weight plateau to give the beast within time to adjust and stop screaming so loudly for more food. Continue with your program, and soon the hunger-related anxiety will settle. You will break through to your next plateau, and the cycle will start again. With each new steady state, you start the discussion with your adipose tissue all over again. Expect this dialog; don't be intimidated by it. Eventually your body figures out that you are not trying to kill it, and it doesn't fight you as much on each step toward your goal. Stick with it, don't rush, remember how long it took to gain the weight, and you'll work through the resistance of the new plateau and achieve success in that fight with the beast.

In Summary

Just as each of the forms of cancer requires its own specialized treatment program, there are many types of excess adipose tissue (obesity), each of which requires its own individualized combination of anti-inflammatory tools—proper diet, good sleep hygiene, exercise, and B vitamers. There is no way to determine ahead of time which combination of tools will work best for you on your curve, so experiment to decide which will become part of your lifestyle.

For dietary folate, look to various meats, beans, lentils, spinach, asparagus, romaine lettuce, and avocado. To ensure that you take in plenty of dietary B12, look to shellfish, eggs, fatty fish, and beef. I know we've long been told to avoid red meat in order to reduce the risk of heart disease, but we're finding out that sugar and carbohydrates are a bigger danger, especially if you eat fresh meat in moderation. There is another way of using B vitamers to actually reduce the need and drive to consume red meat. Anecdotally, my patients have noted a decrease urge to eat red meat when they start daily vitamer supplementation, but more about this in a later chapter.

Now that we have studied the biochemistry of vitamers, the epigenetics of DNA, and the reduction of inflammatory loads by modulators, we can put it all together in the next chapter as we learn how to use vitamers and other tools to build an enduring low inflammatory healthy homeostasis.

ELEVEN

VITAMER THERAPEUTICS— MODULATOR OF MODULATORS

"Normal" Serum B12 in the US ≠ "Normal" in Japan ≠ "Normal" in Australia

Diagnosing a B12 or folate deficiency is not the simple matter most people think it is, because the tests used are inadequate and often misleading. Doctors generally rely on a single test for B12 or folate levels in the blood. This may or may not be an accurate reflection of vitamer availability throughout the body. Blood tests do not always tell us all we need to know about whether the body cells are receiving and able to use the synthetic vitamins taken in. The truth is deficiency-driven symptoms occur in people who have "normal" lab results. The problem begins with the difficulty of finding a physician with the knowledge that a B-vitamin deficiency can be present even in the absence of the classical deficiency test of macrocytic anemia.

Given the tools at our disposal today, diagnosing a vitamer deficiency is much more of an art than a science. Testing results are generally accepted as in the "normal" range, or else "abnormal" defined as above or below that range. Unfortunately, the scale for acceptable serum B12 levels is enormous, varying from 185 pg/ml to 900 pg/ml. The normal number surprisingly depends on the country you live in (more about that later). This is a huge span, with the top number being almost five times greater than the bottom number. To make matters more confusing, it is possible for a person with a B12 level of 200 to be perfectly healthy, as long as her body is extraordinarily adept at handling B12 and she is not experiencing stressors. Yet a second person with exactly the same serum B12 level could be suffering from clear-cut symptoms, while a third person, with a much higher level of B12, might be suffering from a subclinical yet dangerous deficiency with impending permanent nerve damage. In addition, B12 and folate levels fall with age, so the "healthy" results for seniors are different from those of younger individuals. Normal levels for nonpregnant women are less than for those who are pregnant. These problems are compounded by the fact different laboratories use different techniques to measure B12 and folate.

Then there's the problem of getting a test sample that accurately reflects B12 levels *and* activity within in the body. The usual method is to measure the serum B12 level, giving the total amount of vitamer forms A-B12 and M-B12 in the fluid part of the blood, a combination of free-floating B12 plus the active B12 attached to a transporter protein called holo-transcobalamin (holoTC).[115] About 20 to 25 percent of B12 is in this protein-bound active form, which is transported into the cells and across the blood-brain barrier. The remaining 75 percent eventually passes unused out of the body. Because only the active form has any relevance to health, over thirty years ago Dr. Victor Herbert suggested looking at holoTC as a measure of B12 activity. Since then, others have suggested using holo-TC as the initial screening test, and if it is not definitive, then follow up with an MMA (methylmalonic acid) level (see chapter three). But there's no consensus yet, and I imagine most physicians ordering routine B12 tests are not even aware of these issues—I wasn't.

Is "Japanese B12" the Same as "American B12?"

To make the challenge of measuring B12 even more difficult, the "normal" level varies from country to country. In the United States, below 200 pg/mL is the point at which a deficiency diagnosis is made and treatment initiated. It is below 500 pg/mL in Japan, two-and-a-half times higher than the American level and almost four times higher than the Australian level of 135 pg/mL. In Japan the level is set below which nerve dysfunction occurs, while in the US it is set at the level below which anemia appears. In Japan and European countries, the portion of older populations suffering from dementias like Alzheimer's is significantly lower than in the United States. Is this a coincidence? It has been suggested by many physicians (I count myself among them) that we rethink the alarmingly low level that must be reached

115 Hoffmann-Lücke, E., and Nexo, E., "Holotranscobalamin, a Marker of Vitamin B-12 Status: Analytical Aspects and Clinical Utility," *American Journal of Clinical Nutrition*, July 2011; 94(1):359S–365S.

before initiating treatment. Unfortunately, as a researcher pointed out in the *Journal of Internal Medicine*, "It is not unusual that health authorities refuse prescriptions for vitamin B12 in patients with clinical signs of neuropathy because the patients have no haematological signs (abnormal blood values), and their plasma vitamin B12 levels are reported as 'normal.'"[116]

Trouble Testing for Folate

Trying to determine an accurate folate level can be equally confusing, starting with the terminology. A correct serum folate level reflects the actual amount of the active vitamer L-methyl-tetrahydrofolate, the bioactive form the body uses. Physicians typically order folate tests by checking a box on a lab request sheet, where it is often listed as a "folate (folic acid)" test, using the names of the vitamer and artificial forms interchangeably. According to the commercial laboratories I contacted, it is really the folic acid level being tested, and folate has to be requested separately.

While a serum folate test is useful for determining a deficiency, it only measures folate levels at the moment the blood is drawn. A better indicator of long-term folate status is the amount of folate contained in the red blood cells.

Here are the standard folate tests that can be ordered from most national labs:

- Folate, RBC – folate in the red blood cells
- Folate, RBC, and Serum – folate in the red blood cells and serum
- Folate (Folic Acid) – but which is it, folate or folic acid?
- Vitamin B12 and Folates – B12 and various folate forms, but which ones?

This list appears to be comprehensive, but an important issue is raised. It makes no sense to try to understand how the body handles folic acid in supplements and food if there is no awareness of whether the folic acid can even be converted into folate. In other words, what is the status of the MTHFR enzyme? Though this is not usually measured, an understanding of an individual's nutrient status would be incomplete without it. Everyone should know their MTHFR status, most critically if they are planning a pregnancy. My hope is that in the future this status will be noted on medical records just as allergies and blood types are.

---

[116] Smith, A.D., Refsum, H., "Do We Need to Reconsider the Desirable Blood Level of Vitamin B12?" *Journal of Internal Medicine*, 2011; 271(2):179–182.

Surrogate Measures Can Clarify the Matter

Obviously, our standard approach to checking vitamer deficiencies is grossly inadequate. The best approach would be to use various direct and indirect measures to provide as much information as possible about the levels of utilization of the vitamers. Ideally, we would look at the levels in the brain, where B12/folate shortages can cause dementia, stroke, and other disorders. A sample of brain tissue would provide the most definitive answer available, but obtaining the sample requires a procedure most people and their physicians would prefer to skip. The next most accurate approach would be to measure the vitamer levels in the spinal fluid, which would require a spinal tap. This procedure necessitates the insertion of a large needle through the lower back into the spinal canal to withdraw fluid, with its own perils and costs.

The most practical method to determine a B12/F deficiency is to seek evidence of it inside the body's cells by checking the levels of homocysteine and MMA (methylmalonic acid), two metabolic by-products of insufficient B12/folate. As you may remember, a lack of the vitamers causes homocysteine levels to rise. This is true even if folate levels are adequate, because folate cannot "stand in" for B12 when it comes to metabolizing homocysteine and MMA. An elevated MMA level may show up early in the B12 deficit process, but not always.[117]

Measuring homocysteine presents its own challenge, for the patient must stay on a low-protein diet for several days followed by an overnight fast for the most reliable results.

Quick, Accurate, and Pain-Free Blood Test

Optical B12 sensors are a major advancement in diagnosing B12 deficiency. Developed by Dr. Georgios Tsiminis of Melbourne, Australia, the sensor views blood flow through the skin without puncturing it to determine B12 levels. Each molecule viewed through spectroscopy gives off a unique color code. Dr. Tsiminis developed the sensor so physicians could obtain inexpensive and immediate lab results. Perhaps one day this test will become a standard for measuring B12 levels.[118]

---

[117] Hannibal, L., Lysne, V., Bjørke-Monsen, A.L., et al, "Biomarkers and Algorithms for the Diagnosis of Vitamin B12 Deficiency," *Frontiers in Molecular Biosciences*, 2016; 3:27.

[118] Tsiminis, G., et al, "Measurements of Vitamin B12 in Human Blood Serum Using Raman Spectroscopy," presented at *SPIE BioPhotonics Australasia*; Adelaide, Australia, October 16–19, 2016.

Diagnosing a Deficit from All Directions

Since we still lack a single and simple way to measure active B_{12} and folate levels, we must rely on several measures, each providing a peek at the full picture. Here is a list of tests used as a group to get the most accurate picture possible of B_{12} and folate levels and activity:

- *Serum B_{12}* – While this is a starting point, the result rarely provides enough information for an accurate diagnosis by itself.

- *Serum folate* – Measuring folate rather than folic acid is critical. Your physician can specifically request that the lab check folate levels. If serum B_{12} and serum folate tests are both normal, but symptoms seem to indicate deficiency, the following tests on this list should be considered.

- *CBC* – This is a complete blood count measuring the number, content, and appearance of red blood cells, white blood cells, and platelets, and it gives an indication of the presence of anemia or infections. If macrocytic anemia is present, the results of the CBC must be combined with other lab results to rule out causes of macrocytic anemia, including alcoholic liver disease, blood loss, low thyroid function, and medication side effects.

- *Serum iron* – A deficiency of the mineral iron causes iron-deficiency anemia, which can confuse the diagnosis of a B_{12}/folate anemia. The red blood cells seen with iron deficiency anemia are smaller (microcytic anemia) because they have a reduced amount of iron-based hemoglobin molecules. Mixing the macrocytic anemia of B_{12}/F deficiency with the microcytic anemia of iron deficiency can make the cell size look normal, while the cells themselves are significantly abnormal.

- *MTHFR enzyme functioning* – This measures the body's ability to convert folic acid to folate. Reduced MTHFR enzyme function hampers cellular folate production in over 50 percent of people, which is important if you are taking folic acid supplements and rely on the conversion—but not important if you are taking the folate vitamer, which does not need to be converted.

- *MMA* – This test measures B_{12} cellular efficiency, with a high MMA indicating a B_{12} deficiency. While the deficiency sometimes occurs early in the disease process, it may not appear until later on, so this test alone cannot be relied on to diagnose B12 deficiency.

- *Homocysteine* – Elevated homocysteine occurs in B12 and folate deficiency, but also results from alcohol abuse, genetic abnormalities, and renal failure. If there is only a folate deficiency, then homocysteine will be higher, while the MMA will remain within the normal range. If both MMA and homocysteine are normal, a diagnosis of a B12/F deficiency is quite unlikely.

- *Intrinsic factor antibodies* – A positive result indicates the presence of an autoimmune process blocking the stomach's ability to make intrinsic factor, necessary to transport B12 to the small intestine. This causes pernicious anemia that shows up as a macrocytic anemia or simply the neurologic symptoms of a B12 deficiency.

- *Schilling Test* – This test, rarely performed nowadays, uses radioactive labeled B12 to determine whether or not one makes enough intrinsic factor to absorb B12 from food. An inability to manufacture intrinsic factor leads to B12 deficiency and the resulting pernicious anemia.

- *Nerve conduction studies* – B12 deficiency causes a condition called subacute combined degeneration of the coverings of the nerves (the myelin sheath), resulting in weakness, fatigue, balance problems, difficulty walking, and numbness and tingling of the extremities. Measuring the speed at which an electric impulse is conducted along the nerve detects dysfunction in the myelin sheath and the nerve/muscle connections.

Testing for Inflammation

When B12 and folate fall below optimal levels, energy levels drop, the cells fill up with metabolic "trash," and subpar levels of certain proteins are produced. This, in turn, leads to chronic inflammation. While chronic inflammation by itself isn't proof of a B12 or folate deficiency, inflammation that's unrelated to a specific cause, such as a viral infection, is more likely to occur when these two nutrients are in short supply. Fortunately, there are some blood tests indicating the presence of inflammation, including:

- *White blood cell count* – The body pumps out more white blood cells during inflammation as it struggles to right itself. A high level indicates inflammation is present somewhere in the body.

- *Platelet count* – Platelets, found in large numbers in the blood and involved in clotting, help repair internal damage. Their numbers increase when the body is fighting to regain homeostasis.

- *C-reactive protein* (CRP) – CRP is a protein created in response to any kind of inflammatory challenge. It is measured in the form of high-sensitivity-CRP (hs-CRP).

- *Erythrocyte sedimentation rate* – This test measures how quickly red blood cells settle to the bottom of a test tube. If there is an increase in the number of inflammatory proteins on the surface of the cells, they will be heavier and settle to the bottom more quickly.

- *Plasma viscosity* – The more inflammatory protein and homocysteine there is in the serum, the thicker (more viscous) the blood plasma will be and the greater the likelihood of blood-clot formation (thromboemboli).

- *Interleukin-6 (IL-6)* – While the other items on this list are passive indicators of inflammation, interleukin-6 is a pro-inflammatory cytokine that increases with inflammation and by itself worsens inflammation. Manufactured by the white blood cells as well as adipose tissue, IL-6 stimulates the production of more white blood cells and other interleukins, causing an even greater inflammatory response over time and accelerating the unhealthy aging process. The IL-6 cytokine is perhaps the single best test to monitor for signs of inflammation.

Given the difficult of pinpointing B12 and folate levels and usage in the body with the standard blood test, it makes sense to keep all these tests in mind when working toward a diagnosis. And, of course, your doctor must also factor in your clinical presentation, diet, personal habits, and medications, as well as any increased risk of deficiency due to pregnancy, Crohn's disease, autoimmune illnesses, celiac disease, HIV, or other conditions.

Vitamer Supplementation: Buyer Beware!

For the sake of discussion, let's say you've been diagnosed with a deficiency of B12, folate, or both. Your physician recommends supplementation to restore optimal levels. She suggests an over-the-counter form of B12 and/or folate or prescribes one of the higher dose forms.

Until fairly recently, it was difficult to get the vitamer folate in either prescription or over-the counter (OTC) form, for the folate molecule is not stable and has a short shelf life. Around the year 2000, a new biochemical process was developed that extended the vitamers' shelf life enough so they could be provided in supplement form. Theoretically, this meant everyone now had a choice—they could take folate supplements instead of the possibly useless, man-made folic acid.

Unfortunately, the labels on many supplement bottles do not accurately reflect what's actually inside the pills, especially if the supplements are made in countries with even fewer regulations than we have in the United States. While many of these folate supplements claim that they consist of L-methylfolate, they are actually in a form not able to be used by the body.

A Thousand a Day Is the Way

The OTC dose of folate available without prescription is regulated by the government. A dose of 1 milligram (1000 micrograms) per day has been chosen by the FDA as the maximum amount available without a doctor's prescription. This amount, it turns out, is probably the minimal optimal daily dose of L-methylfolate to aid healthy living for most individuals.

Higher Percentage Requires Rx

Many supplements and medications have similar FDA concentrations restrictions. Lower doses are available OTC, but higher concentrations require a prescription. As an example, hydrocortisone cream for allergic reactions is sold over the counter at 1 percent concentration, while 2.5 percent concentration requires a prescription.

There is no upper limit for B12 sold over the counter because the vitamer has a large safety profile, even with high doses. I recommend to my patients that the B12 taken should always be in the vitamer form, either as A-B12 (adenosylcobalamin) and/or M-B12 (methylcobalamin) in a total daily dose of at least 2 mg (2,000 mcg) per day. B12 and folate should always be taken together to bypass the possibility that taking only one might miss a deficiency of the other.

Folic Acid Fallacy

Back in the late 1940s, it was thought that folic acid used to treat anemia would worsen the neuropathy caused by an undiagnosed B12 deficiency. This lack of knowledge was incorporated into guidelines for a prescribing upper limit on folic acid in 1998 when grain fortification became mandatory in the US. This false foundation has been used to limit folic acid consumption and to prevent the voluntary fortification of grains in many countries, to the detriment to of public health and medical costs.[119]

Let's assume the mandatory Supplemental Facts Label found on a supplement bottle is absolutely accurate. Still, you must read the label to understand what is contained in the pill, keeping in mind that it does not tell you how much of each ingredient will end up in the form of bioactive vitamers in your body. Pay attention to what's on the entire Supplement Facts label, including the list of "ingredients" toward the bottom, where you may discover the real kind of vitamins used and the fillers added. For example, the label from a popular vitamin brand (shown below) indicates the folate is actually folic acid, while the B12 is in the cyano form:

Supplement Facts

Serving Size: 1 Tablet   Servings Per Container: 30

	Amount Per Tablet	% Daily Value
Vitamin B6 (as pyridoxine HCl)	5 mg	250%
Folate (as folic acid)	400 mcg	100%
Vitamin B12 (cyanocobalamin)	1000 mcg	16,667%
Biotin	25 mcg	8%

The information on the next label is a bit cloudier, as the forms of B12 and folate are not revealed. You can't tell if you are getting helpful vitamer form or the sometimes-useless vitamin form. You can see they are derived from a yeast culture, although this culture may contain other vitamins used by yeasts but not by humans.

---

[119] Berry, R.J., "Lack of Historical Evidence to Support Folic Acid Exacerbation of the Neuropathy Caused by Vitamin B12 Deficiency," *American Journal of Clinical Nutrition*. September 1, 2019; 110(3):554–561.

SUPPLEMENT FACTS

Serving Size: 1 Tablets
Serving per Container: 60

Amount per Serving		% Daily Value
Thiamine (from Saccharomyces Cerevisiae)	2 mg	133%
Riboflavin (from Saccharomyces Cerevisiae)	3 mg	176%
Niacin (as Niacinamide) (from Saccharomyces Cerevisiae)	20 mg	100%
Vitamin B6 (from Saccharomyces Cerevisiae)	9 mg	450%
Folate (from Saccharomyces Cerevisiae)	250 mcg	63%
Vitamin B12 (from Saccharomyces Cerevisiae)	200mcg	3333%

When deciphering other labels, such as the one below, you need to study the ingredients in order to find out that B12 is in the form of cyanocobalamin and folic acid is in the form of folinic acid, which is the "in-between" folate form.

Folic Acid	200 mcg	50 %
Vitamin B-12	6 mcg	100 %
Trimethylglycine (HCL)	175 mg	**

* Percent Daily Values Based on a 2000 calorie diet.
** Daily Value Not Established.

INGREDIENTS: Trimethylglycine, MicroCrystalline Cellulose, Folinic Acid, Magnesium Stearate (vegetable), Silicon Dioxide, Cyanocobalamin, Plant Cellulose Capsule.

Yet Another Form of Folate

Folinic acid, also known as 5-formyl tetrahydrofolate, is halfway between folic acid and folate. Folinic acid doesn't have to be metabolized by the liver as much as folic acid does to be converted it into folate, but it still requires the MTHFR enzyme in the final step to form 5-L-methyltetrahydrofolate. This is not good or bad as much as a half-step to where you should be.

Glancing at the next supplement label, you can see that the multivitamin/ multi-mineral tablet is crammed with nineteen ingredients. It's hard to imagine they all have been handled with care and that each will properly separate from the others in the intestines and be absorbed and metabolized into the bioactive vitamins and minerals the body uses.

Amount Per Serving		% Daily Value
Vitamin A (as retinyl acetate, beta-carotene)	10,000IU	200%
Vitamin C (as ascorbic acid, calcium ascorbate)	135mg	225%
Vitamin D as cholecalciferol)	400IU	100%
Vitamin E (as dl-alpha tocopheryl acetate, d-alpha tocopheryl acetate)	90IU	300%
Thiamin (as thiamin mononitrate)	20mg	1,333%
Riboflavin	13.5mg	794%
Niacin (as niacinamide, nicotinic acid)	60mg	300%
Vitamin B6 (as pyridoxine hydrochloride, pyridoxal-5-phosphate)	10mg	500%
Folic acid	300mcg	75%
Vitamin B12 (as cyanocobalamin)	100mcg	1667%
Biotin	165mcg	55%
Pantothenic acid (as calcium d-pantothenate)	80mg	800%
Calcium (as calcium carbonate, calcium citrate)	152mg	15%
Magnesium (as magnesium oxide)	145mg	36%
Zinc (as zinc oxide, zinc amino acid chelate)	9.5mg	63%
Copper (as copper amino acid chelate)	1mg	50%
Manganese (as manganese sulfate monohydrate)	7mg	350%
Molybdenum (as molybdenum amino acid chelate)	10mcg	13%
Potassium (as potassium chloride)	35mg	1%

You might think the FDA would ensure that all vitamins—at least all American-made ones—contain the vitamer forms and are prepared in such a way the body can fully absorb each ingredient. While it is true that the FDA issues guidelines called Good Manufacturing Practices for the production of supplements, it does not monitor each and every manufacturing site in the country, let alone around the world. This unsupervised production allows for contaminants, inactive ingredients, ingredients not listed on the label, doses lower or higher than noted, and other problems. Some brands have been contaminated with steroids, antidepressants, and male sexual enhancers. Even after contaminants are discovered and a recall has been issued, some bottles may remain on the shelves for years.[120]

The FDA also maintains guidelines called Good Distribution Practices to ensure the proper shipping, storage, and distribution of over-the-counter and prescribed pharmaceuticals. Like the other guidelines, they are not foolproof. My best advice is this: buyer beware. It is best to buy a brand from a reputable manufacturer, but only after researching that brand. Log onto www.ConsumerLab.com, where you will find the results of tests conducted on many brands using supplements taken off the shelf in stores, rather than bottles provided by the manufacturer. One of ConsumerLab's studies examined forty-five different brands of multivitamins. Fifteen (one-third) of

---

[120] Cohen, P.A., "Presence of Banned Drugs in Dietary Supplements Following FDA Recalls," *Journal of the American Medical Association*, 2014; 312(16):1691–1693.

these were not approved by ConsumerLab because they contained lower or higher doses than stated on the label, or ingredients that were not listed on the label at all.

It amazes me that people will buy a four-dollar cup of coffee every day but refuse to pay more than pennies for a daily vitamin that actually works.

Injection Selection

For the sake of discussion, let's say you have a severe depletion of B12. Your doctor recommends intramuscular B12 injections, saying they will bypass any problems with absorption. If the C-B12 or the H-B12 forms are used, they must still cycle through the liver several times before being converted into bioactive vitamers. Injected M-B12 or A-B12 bioactivity will still be limited by the amount of transporter protein you have available to take the B12 from the injection site into the cells.

Is it worthwhile to use injections instead of oral supplements? In general, if you follow the oral dosing schedule carefully, there seems to be little practical difference in the initial use with either form. If one of my patients had serious symptoms of a deficiency, I would probably recommend starting with injections for a quick "bump up," then follow up with an oral schedule.

Injections are usually beneficial, but typically too much is given in one shot. If the shot is in the vitamin form, this single high dose overwhelms the body's ability to convert the vitamins into vitamers, and there are not enough transporter proteins available to pull the vitamers into the cells. If the shot is in the bioactive form, a large dose also overwhelms the carrier proteins, but it is absorbed into the cells so rapidly that a lot more gets captured compared to the synthetic vitamins. If a patient is in critical need, several lower-dose intramuscular injections over a week would be more beneficial. Sublingual doses bypass the liver on the first cycle of the blood circulation, which slows down the ability of the liver to convert the artificial forms into vitamers. The benefits, or lack thereof, are the same as oral doses.

Taking Your Vitamer Supplements

Let's say you've found a vitamer supplement offering the right dose. It was made by a reputable manufacturer and has been carefully stored away from light and humidity. You are finally ready take it, but if you do not ingest it correctly, all will be for naught.

The most important rule in using vitamers is to take them on an empty stomach, with four ounces of water—and only water. The four ounces are necessary to fully dissolve the tablet and dilute the ingredients for efficient absorption. Remember, the vitamers are sensitive to the presence of other vitamins and minerals (iron), as well as vitamin C in juice, and will bind up and become useless in their presence. So take your vitamers by themselves, without other supplements or food. You can still take your multivitamin supplement with meals, for any possible benefit, as long as it doesn't have a lot of folic acid that might block the absorption of folate vitamers into the brain.

Remember, however, vitamer supplements cannot make up for poor nutrition. If your food is not of the right quality and variety, your health will suffer. And it's important to bear in mind that the use of vitamers is not intended to *treat* medical conditions such as diabetes, heart disease, or depression. The vitamers should only be used as adjuncts to facilitate other treatments prescribed by your physician. Some populations with a B_{12}/F deficiency and medical conditions such as pregnancy, HIV, anorexia, and post-operative recovery, might need the higher prescription doses just to catch up to "normal" before switching to an over-the-counter dose for maintenance.

I typically tell my patients to try the vitamers for three months and continue if they see improvements. If they do not notice any benefits, I tell them to stop taking the supplements for three to four weeks. As with certain other medications, sometimes you don't realize how much it has helped until you stop. Occasionally, you won't notice the benefits, but your friends and family will. For example, they are often better able than you are to detect subtle positive changes in your mood, speech, and memory.

Sometimes with a "vitamer assist," you feel the change and sometimes even see a change. The first thing many of my patients who responded to vitamers noticed was thicker nails and hair and skin injuries that healed more quickly.

Keep in mind that over-diagnosing people with a deficiency has little downside, as treatment with folate or B_{12} has few, if any, hazards, while underdiagnosis has serious consequences of permanent nerve damage, heart disease, and dementias. There are some unique medical situations requiring specific dosing for B_{12} or folate. For example, if someone is taking methotrexate as chemotherapy, they should consult with their physician before supplementing with folate. As mentioned before, it is vital to always make sure your physicians know about all supplementation used.

The Evidence Is Fishy

Fish oil supplements are often touted as being anti-inflammatory. While some studies are intriguing, there is no convincing evidence of the advantages of fish oil beyond possible blood-thinning benefits.[121] Meanwhile, catching all the fish necessary to fill those fish oil capsules so many people swallow is destroying the ecosystem of the oceans, wiping out foundational fish low on the food chain. It is these fish that support the health of the ocean food cycle upon which the rest of the world relies for its vitamer source. If fish oil is at best no better than other thinning agents like aspirin, then the cost of fish oil supplements to our planet's future far outweighs their questionable benefits.

Prescribed and OTC Meds That Block or Deplete B Vitamins

There is a significant number of prescribed and OTC medications that deplete or block the use of B vitamins. If you are taking one of these, it is important that your physician is aware of and recommends a vitamer supplement. Below is a partial list of the categories.

- *Antacids* – cimetidine, famotidine, ranitidine, lansoprazole, nizatidine, omeprazole
- *Anti-inflammatory treatments* – prednisone
- *Anti-Parkinson's medication* – carbidopa, levodopa
- *Antibiotics* – trimethoprim, sulfa derivatives, penicillin
- *Anticonvulsants* – carbamazepine, ethosuximide, phenobarbital, phenytoin, valproic acid
- *Anti-diabetic medications* – metformin
- *Asthma medications* – oral/nasal inhalers beclomethasone, budesonide, fluticasone
- *Blood pressure medication* – bumetanide, hydrochlorothiazide, furosemide, hydralazine
- *Cholesterol reduction medication* – cholestyramine, statins

---

[121] Manson, JoAnn E., "Marine n–3 Fatty Acids and Prevention of Cardiovascular Disease and Cancer," *New England Journal of Medicine*, January 3, 2019; 380:23–32.

- *Estrogen/ estrogen substitutes* – estrogen with or w/o progesterone (BCP, HRT), raloxifene

- *Pain treatment* – aspirin and aspirin containing products

- *Nonsteroidal anti-inflammatory drugs* – naproxen, indomethacin, celecoxib, ibuprofen

A Final Word

A final point on labels. To interpret a true "% daily value," remember, only 1% of B_{12} is absorbed by passive diffusion so the percentages on the labels are way off. They assume 100% absorption of 1,000 mcg to get their super high inaccurate "% daily value" of 16,667%. If a tablet has 1000 mcg, that means 10 micrograms absorbed at most. If the body needs 2.4 mcg of B_{12} per day, then the actual percentage is at most 417% (1000/2.4), not 16,667%.

One of the nicest things about B_{12} and folate is they work well with almost every medical treatment. They also work with any modulator you have chosen to improve your health, be it exercise, meditation, dietary changes, or something else. The vitamers are a sort of "universal optimizing agent," strengthening you and improving your odds of enjoying better health, no matter what your current state. Taking bioactive vitamins daily is a form of health insurance. I certainly hope you maximize your modulators and do all you can to ensure a longer, healthier life.

TWELVE

PUTTING IT ALL TOGETHER

↑Stressors→↑Stress→↓Functioning→
↑Inflammatory Load →Unhealthy Aging

We've tackled some rather complex subjects in our quest to understand the vital role of the vitamers. We have learned:

- The body uses vitamers B12 and folate to create energy, cleanse the cells of waste products, and modulate the expression of genes.

- An insufficient supply of these B-vitamers hampers these critical functions and thereby increases the body's inflammatory load, among other problems.

- As the inflammatory load increases, the risk of developing an inflammatory-based illness such as cardiovascular disease rises.

- Increased inflammation contributes to nine out of ten leading causes of illness and death in the United States.

- The degree to which you are likely to develop an inflammation-driven illness is influenced by the many factors making up your lens (stressors focused into stress responses).

- All modulators reducing your inflammatory load depend on the presence of ample amounts of vitamers B12 and folate for maximum effectiveness.

Vitamers Prevent Inflammation-Based Illness

Putting all this together, we can say that one or more stressors upsetting homeostasis and triggering inflammation is the "universal illness," the underlying cause of most of our fatal ailments. The vitamers are the "spark plugs" supercharging the body's battle against inflammation and making it possible for all other anti-inflammatory steps to be maximally effective. These precious nutrients must be present in ample amounts for other measures to work well. The body may start reacting with a perfectly normal and healthy inflammatory response, followed by an increased inflammatory load and chronic inflammation that leads to the dreaded diseases ruining far too many lives.

Medical science is well aware of the devastating effects of inflammation on human health. Unfortunately, you will not find reams of research on the reduction of inflammation with B vitamers because there is little profit from this simple, inexpensive intervention. Pharmaceutical and medical device companies make huge profits treating the aftereffects of inflammation, so that is where their focus remains. New studies need to be conducted on the benefits of vitamers, and all earlier studies using artificial supplements previously showing equivocal results should be repeated with vitamers.

We do have smaller, short-term studies on B-supplement treatment for inflammation-related illnesses. Unfortunately, most of these studies fail to note the form of B12 used and often use "folate" to mean "folic acid," which is misleading. Were the vitamers used, or was it the man-made form? It is not clear. Even when the vitamers or vitamins are properly noted, they are usually administered in inadequate doses. Making matters worse, B12 and folate are often evaluated singly in research studies, not as the "partner nutrients" they are. Since either vitamer is weaker on its own, it is easy for researchers testing them one at a time to conclude they are less effective. Yet another problem is that most of supplement efficacy studies use subjects who *already have* a clinical illness. Often, they have already incurred serious and irreversible damage, making it impossible to restore them to ideal health and leading researchers to conclude the B-vitamins or vitamers are not effective.

Lacking the long-term, large-scale studies we need and relying on existing poorly designed short-term studies, we must extrapolate from the research conducted using the manufactured forms of C-B12 and folic acid. If these inefficient forms help against the major illnesses of inflammation, then the natural bioactive forms should be even more beneficial.

With these limitations, scientific studies do demonstrate that even B's in the vitamin form can be helpful in the battle against inflammation-based diseases. We've already reviewed a number of studies; here are a few more:

- *Dementia* – Australian researchers found that when B vitamins are given to treat the cognitive decline preceding dementia, there is a positive benefit in cognitive function after twenty-four months.[122] This study was done with folic acid and an undisclosed form of B12.

- *Breast cancer* – Like the previous study, this one showed that B-vitamins slowed the progression of an illness—in this case, breast cancer. In this study, researchers from Harvard and Tufts found that higher blood levels of folate may reduce the risk of developing breast cancer. Especially among women consuming at least 15 grams of alcohol daily, higher levels of plasma folate were associated with lower risk of breast cancer. Higher levels of plasma B12 were also associated with a lower risk of breast cancer among premenopausal women.[123]

- *Stroke* – The researchers followed over forty thousand men, ages forty to seventy-five, for fourteen years to track the effects of B-vitamins on the risk of suffering a stroke. They found that incidence of stroke caused by arterial blockage decreased with increased intake of folic acid and B12.[124] This study did not use folate or note the kind of B12 used.

- *Diabetes mellitus* – A placebo-controlled, multicenter study using a prescription formulation of methylcobalamin and folate found that these B vitamers reduced the symptoms of diabetic neuropathy.[125]

Almost all of the current studies on the benefit of B-vitamins have been performed using the manufactured forms, not the vitamer forms.

---

[122] Walker, J.G., Batterham, P.J., Mackinnon, A.J., et al, "Oral Folic Acid and Vitamin B-12 Supplementation to Prevent Cognitive Decline in Community-Dwelling Older Adults with Depressive Symptoms—The Beyond Ageing Project: A Randomized Controlled Trial," *American Journal of Clinical Nutrition*, 2012; 95(1):194–203.

[123] Zhang, S.M., Willet, W.C., Selhub, J., et al, "Plasma Folate, Vitamin B6, Vitamin B12, Homocysteine, and Risk of Breast Cancer," *Journal of the National Cancer Institute*, 2003; 95(5):373–380.

[124] Ka, He, Merchant, A., Rimm, E.B., et al, "Folate, Vitamin B6, and B12 Intakes in Relation to Risk of Stroke Among Men, *Stroke*, 2004; 35:169–174.

[125] Fonseca, V.A., "Metanx in Type 2 Diabetes with Peripheral Neuropathy: A Randomized Trial," *American Journal of Medicine*, 2013; 126(2):141–9.

This makes me wish for powerful studies examining the ability of the B-vitamers to reduce much of the suffering of inflammation-related illnesses.

Graphing Your Wave

Throughout the book, we've talked about the slide from health to illness as if it occurred in a straight-line manner: first this happens, then that, and so on. That's not necessarily how it occurs in real life, where the progression from good health to bad is more often like a roller coaster ride, with ups and downs—sometimes big ones—eventually leaving you at a lower level of functioning than when you began. For other people, however, the ride is relatively smooth and leaves them pretty much where they began.

To help patients understand this, I often draw a wavy-line graph to illustrate how they might have arrived at their current state. The wavy-line graph shows where they were before the stressor hit and how their health varies on a daily, monthly, and even yearly basis.

For example, as you see in figure 1, a hypothetical patient's health trends up and down on a regular basis. Even when he's in great health, there will be some variation, some highs and lows, as he absorbs the shocks and stresses of living, is exposed to bacteria and unpleasant people, rides out bad times at work, falters a bit when injured, and shines when he takes good care of himself. The inflammatory load increases a bit with each downturn, then recedes a bit with each upturn.

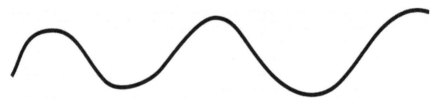

Figure 1

Occasionally, the patient's "health wave" takes a greater dip (figure 2), which may last a day, a week, a month, or longer. Fortunately, most people bounce back, and their waves return to the stable position they have maintained for years. If this patient's stress is significant—for example, if he goes through a divorce—the downturn will be greater and last longer, with a slower return to the previously normal range.

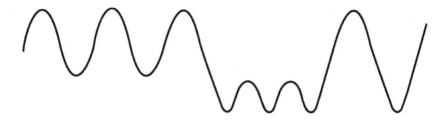

Figure 2

On the positive side, when he has a good phase, his waves trend higher. Perhaps he received a promotion or began a new relationship (figure 3).

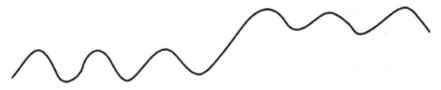

Figure 3

Most of us hold steady for long periods of time on this wavy-line graph, trending up and down in a certain range. If you remain in a higher range— say, in the nineties on a scale of zero to one hundred—you feel great. And even if the range is lower, let's say in the seventies or sixties, you probably feel at least OK because things are in a steady state and there are no obvious or overwhelming symptoms to alarm you.

Even though you may feel OK, where you happen to be trending on the graph at any given time matters. This is your starting point, or as I describe it, your *degree of predisposition.* The lower on the scale, the greater your degree of predisposition and the more inclined you will be toward dropping further down on the scale and developing a physical or psychological illness, whether it's depression, diabetes, dementia, cancer, or something equally devastating.

Apply the idea of a degree of predisposition to the likelihood of a woman developing skin cancer: If she was born with darker skin, providing some protection against skin cancer, her starting range may be in the nineties. If she has fair skin, her range will be lower. Let's say she has fair skin and her baseline is in the seventies. If she suffered several severe sunburns as a child, her baseline will drop even lower, perhaps into the sixties. This new level of predisposition puts her fairly close to the fifty-point line which, solely for the purposes of our one-disease discussion, marks the point where precancerous lesions begin to form. At sixty on our graph, it won't take much of an additional stressor any time in her life to drop her below that line.

While it's great to be perched high on the scale, it's still completely possible to slide into physical illness and mental distress. Indeed, I've seen this happen many times to people, even when they hadn't suffered a catastrophic illness or an emotional blow that might explain such a fall. Instead, there was usually a progression, a series of downward steps triggered by milder physical or emotional stressors. Each factor added to the inflammatory load and made it much harder to achieve recovery.

Putting Numbers to Your Wave

Medical science has yet to create a specific universal blood test with a numeric result showing precisely how healthy or unhealthy a person is. We do have a Global Assessment of Functioning (GAF) scale, used to describe the degree to which someone's mental health is under stress in their daily lives. We will apply this numerical scale to both physical and psychological predispositions, keeping in mind these numbers are not hard and fast, for the GAF is a subjective scale. The scale does serve as a useful tool to understand the levels that can make up a person's predispositions, lens, and modulators. I am using this scale to provide a framework into which we can plug in any ailment. Here is the Global Assessment of Function scale for social health:

Code	Description of Functioning
91 - 100	Person has **no problems** OR has superior functioning in several areas OR is admired and sought after by others due to positive qualities
81 - 90	Person has **few or no symptoms**. Good functioning in several areas. No more than "everyday" problems or concerns.
71 - 80	Person has symptoms/problems, but they are **temporary, expectable reactions to stressors**. There is no more than slight impairment in any area of psychological functioning.
61 - 70	**Mild symptoms in one area** OR difficulty in one of the following: social, occupational, or school functioning. BUT, the person is generally functioning pretty well and has some meaningful interpersonal relationships.
51 - 60	**Moderate symptoms** OR moderate difficulty in one of the following: social, occupational, or school functioning.
41 - 50	**Serious symptoms** OR serious impairment in one of the following: social, occupational, or school functioning.
31 - 40	**Some impairment in reality testing** OR impairment in speech and communication OR serious impairment in several of the following: occupational or school functioning, interpersonal relationships, judgment, thinking, or mood.
21 - 30	Presence of **hallucinations or delusions** which influence behavior OR serious impairment in ability to communicate with others OR serious impairment in judgment OR inability to function in almost all areas.
11 - 20	There is **some danger of harm to self or others** OR occasional failure to maintain personal hygiene OR the person is virtually unable to communicate with others due to being incoherent or mute.
1 - 10	**Persistent danger of harming self or others** OR persistent inability to maintain personal hygiene OR person has made a serious attempt at suicide.

Global Assessment of Functioning (GAF)

Let's apply the GAF concept by adding some numbers to my wavy lines. Remember, these numbers are arbitrarily selected and not meant to suggest that someone is healthy or sick at a certain number. It's simply a way to put the peaks and valleys into perspective. In figure 4 you see a wavy line up around ninety. When a patient is trending around in this range, it means he has excellent health and is simply dealing with the ups and downs of life— the physical injuries, bacterial exposures, psychological stresses, and other problems he cannot avoid. He quickly bounces back from stresses of any sort and remains in good health, with his inflammation load holding at a low level.

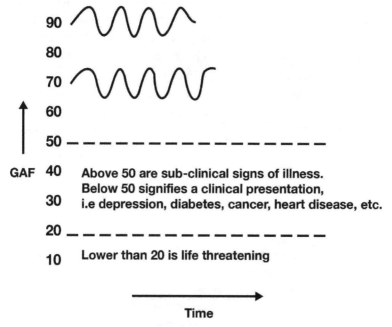

Figure 4

Next, take a look at the wavy line around seventy. At this level, the patient is not as healthy as she would like to be but still functions well. Her inflammatory load is a bit greater than it should be, but it's not pushing her down into the illness region.

Any wavy line below fifty can be defined as poor health. Even if the patient is holding steady at this level, he is not in the best of health. He is at risk of illness should he be hit by a major stress, or even a couple of minor ones. His inflammatory load is slowly undermining the integrity of his arteries and nerves and setting the stage for serious trouble.

As you see in figure 5, another patient is going through her curve and is on a slight upturn because she got a new job. The problem is that it is a change to the night shift with little time for healthy nutritional intake. Her diet suffers and her curve, her level of functioning drops, then she fights back up some. With her poor diet, she develops a vitamer deficiency, and her curve drops again. She again fights back some, never getting as high as before. Then the next stressor occurs—poor sleep from her work cycle resulting in another drop. She claws her way back and feels a little better. The lack of vitamers, sleep, and nutrition, however, exhausts her, and she gives up exercise and socializing, resulting in another drop. Needless to say, her work is now going badly and all her relationships start to suffer, increasing her stress and worsening her functioning. She struggles her way up a little, but the next stressor and the next continue to pull her functioning down until she is so low that she is not functioning at all.

The point being, where we are in our predisposition-to-illness-curve depends on many factors and many stressors that occur just because we are human. It's usually not just one that is the cause of drifting down into inflammation and illness.

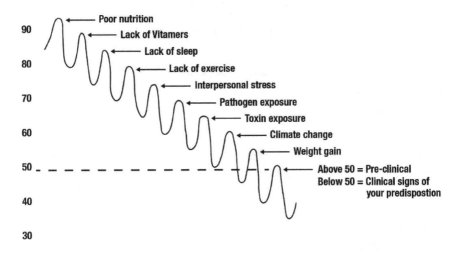

Figure 5

Now let's apply some real-life stressors to another common scenario and the two ways people can respond. Let's say something stressful happens to a woman; for example, her marriage is being dissolved. She was doing fine, but then disagreements began and her curve starts to turn down. On the way down, the divorce is filed, becoming another huge stressor, and her curve drops even more. If she happens to be in the ninety range when subjected to this significant stressor, she might drop down thirty points to the sixty range (figure 6). Her inflammatory load increases and she notices some physical or psychological changes. She might just feel "blah," a bit depressed, or develop some identifiable ailments. She's still above the fifty range, and with work she can probably move back up to the nineties.

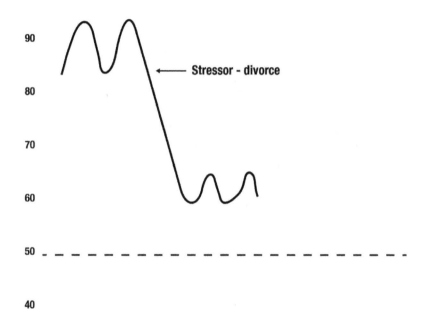

90

80

70

60

50

40

Stressor - divorce

Figure 6

Suppose she began in the seventy range before dropping thirty points. Now she's grinding through her days in the forty range, and her health is at serious risk (figure 7). She probably has developed a diagnosable illness, physical or psychological, and her doctor sternly urges her to use modulators to ease her out of this decline. The modulators might include psychotherapy and psychotropic medication in the short term to speed up the rebound.

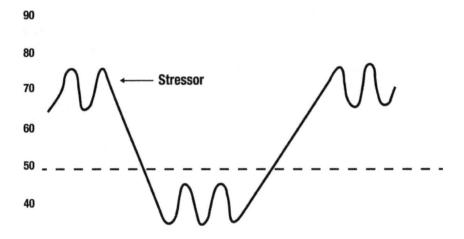

Figure 7

How can she work her way back to better health, and what happens if she doesn't do it? Let's call her Patient A and compare her to Patient B. Both patients begin with a wavy line in the ninety range. Then each gets divorced, and their global functioning plummets into the sixty range. Patient A, whose path is traced in figure 8, begins taking vitamers, exercising, making sure she gets a good night's sleep, sees a therapist, improves her interpersonal skills, limits self-medication (alcohol, cigarettes, narcotics), and otherwise takes good care of herself.

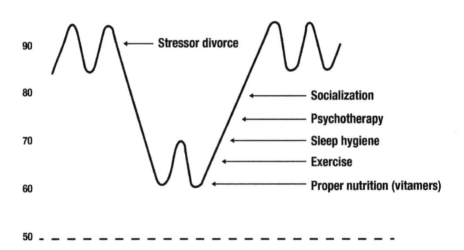

Figure 8

The modulators are each one piece of the puzzle. No single piece turns the tide, but together they are powerful "medicine." Without ample supplies of B12 and folate to generate energy, regulate genetic expression, and keep the cells clear of metabolic waste, all other efforts to improve health will be of reduced benefit.

Compare her to Patient B, whose path is traced in figure 9. This man goes in a totally different direction, self-medicating, declining to exercise, eating poorly, skipping therapy, and not taking B vitamers. Patient B may struggle for years and still not return to his previous level of functioning. Meanwhile, his stress and poor habits ratchet up his inflammatory load and push him into unhealthy aging and quite possibly a fatal illness.

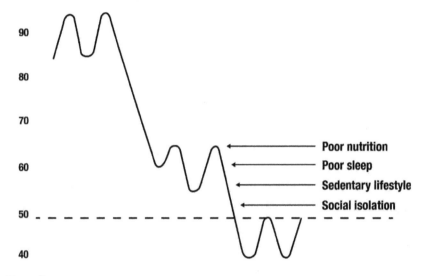

Figure 9

In Summary

There is a never-ending battle raging inside your body, a constant push-and-pull between the stressors raising your inflammatory load and the positive inputs lowering it. Sometimes the battle directly increases the inflammatory load, as when you pack on the extra abdominal fat contributing to inflammation. Sometimes the increase comes about indirectly, as when you weaken the anti-inflammatory modulators by taking certain medicines. You can think of this constant battle like being in a boat bobbing on the ocean. You'll always have to deal with the waves tossing you about and occasionally threatening to crash on your head. You can't stop the waves, but you can do your best to ensure that your boat has as few leaks as possible, your hatches are battened down, and the water is bailed out when taken on.

The stressors of life will continue to wash over you, threatening to overturn your health. The more you use modulators to shift your well-being to a higher level of functioning, the more quickly and efficiently your body will respond to stressors, and the smoother and healthier your sailing through life will be.

THIRTEEN

VITAMERS INTO THE FUTURE—AND BEYOND

↑Vitamers→↓Meat Consumption→
↑Personal and Planetary Health

Vitamers B12 and folate are essential to the health of each and every cell in your body, improving their ability to generate energy, reproduce, cleanse themselves, and share information with one another. When cells are clean, communicating, and producing optimal amounts of energy, body-wide inflammation falls to a low level—enough to maintain good health, but not enough to challenge it. New cells are generated; old ones die off and are absorbed. Time passes at a normal speed, but the body ages at a slower rate and healthily, as it should.

It was thanks to the B vitamers that prehumans emerged so many millions of years ago, and it was thanks to the B vitamers that we were saved from extinction when a climate crisis hit 100,000 years ago. At the same time that our Earth is becoming increasingly crowded and the need for sustenance and arable land increases, scientists are envisioning future missions to Mars. If this exploration is to move forward, it is vital that we never forget we evolved as vitamer-dependent organisms.

Interplanetary Nutrition: Scurvy, Redux?

Aboard Friendship 7, in 1962: The first American to go into orbit, John Glenn, remains in space for five hours as he circles the globe three times. He eats applesauce squeezed out of a tube—not because he's terribly hungry, but rather to see whether it's possible for a human to swallow in the weightlessness of outer space.

Aboard Apollo 11, in 1969: The first men to walk on the moon, led by Neil Armstrong, remain in outer space for 195 hours, or just over eight days. Like other astronauts of the era, they eat freeze-dried, dehydrated, and "thermo-stabilized" foods. Their meals don't look much like real food and aren't very tasty, but they can at least be eaten in weightlessness, with a spoon and without crumbling into a mess.

Aboard the International Space Station today, crew members from various nations remain in space for six months or longer, enjoying a mix of dehydrated, radiated, and "real" foods, plus liquefied salt and pepper.

As we contemplate sending explorers to Mars, missions lasting between one and three years are being planned. Everyone understands that long-distance space travel depends on a deep understanding and application of physics, material science, and many other branches of knowledge. Rocket scientists research these areas to the nth degree, testing and tinkering until nearly the last moment to make things just right. They know from experience that all it takes is a single faulty O-ring or heat tile to trigger a complete disaster.

Although the ramifications of the lunch menu are not nearly as dramatic as failing O-rings, long-distance space travel depends as much on the health of the crew as it does on rocket science. That health depends on optimal nutrition. For example, you wouldn't want someone who has a hidden propensity for illness due to vitamin deficiency to be sent out on a two-year or ten-year mission. The problem might take a year to manifest, but once the rocket ship has blasted off, travelers only turn to what's been brought along. If the problem has to do with vitamer B_{12} or folate, for example, and all there is in the spaceship's medicine chest is standard C-B_{12} and folic acid, trouble could result.

Physical problems caused by nutrient deficiencies would include the fatigue of anemia, nerve damage, thromboemboli, and inefficient inflammatory responses. However, the first symptoms afflicting long-distance travelers would be subtle changes in mood and cognitive function. The affected individuals would be more susceptible to depression, anxiety, memory problems, and decreased reaction times, all while confined in a small space with several other people, some of whom might be suffering from their own deficiency-driven problems.

So far, what's been learned about space nutrition is not encouraging. Despite the culinary improvements, all astronauts lose weight and muscle mass in space. Studies have shown that one out of five astronauts who have spent time on the International Space Station have experienced vision changes upon return to Earth. At first, it was thought this was because of a shift in cranial fluids due to the effect of weightlessness, but this does not explain why a majority of astronauts exposed to microgravity are not likewise affected. Could there be a nutritional component to the problem? A study called the "Nutrition Status Assessment" zeroed in on the blood and urine of space travelers, leading to the discovery that the astronauts whose eyesight worsened had B12 and folate-dependent metabolism abnormalities.[126] If this issue is not addressed, the brave volunteers who make it to Mars might not be able to see well enough to get back.

Another study on the effects of deep space travel, conducted by Dr. Michael Delp at Florida State University, looked at the causes of death of all individuals who had previously participated in the astronaut program.[127] He found those who went into deep space had an astounding 500 percent increase in death due to heart disease compared to controls—that is, the astronauts who only went into low-earth orbit or never got into space at all.

An additional space travel concern recently developed in an unidentified astronaut stationed on the space station. During a routine medical experiment, it was discovered he had developed an obstructive jugular-vein thrombosis.[128] He was successfully treated on board, making a full recovery upon return, but the question raised was how to improve approaches toward prevention. I would suggest that a B12/F deficiency might have caused an increase in homocysteine that would increase blood viscosity in susceptible individuals. The causes could be genetic (↓MTHFR), medication side effects, onboard dietary deficiencies, or supplement failure. A complete blood screen, genetic testing, and supplement review for these vulnerabilities should be initiated for all space travelers.

Humans traveling outside the protective envelope of Earth's magnetic field are exposed to the background radiation of space. It is thought that radiation exposure of any kind causes a chronic inflammatory response in tissue cells, particularly those of the heart vessels. Perhaps this explains the increase in heart disease among high-flying astronauts. To test this hypothesis, a follow-up study was performed on mice who were exposed to the same radiation levels

---

[126] Zwart, S.R., Gibson, C.R., Mader, T.H., et al, "Vision Changes after Spaceflight Are Related to Alterations in Folate—and Vitamin B-12—Dependent One-Carbon Metabolism," *Journal of Nutrition*, 2012; 142(3):427–431.

[127] Delp, M., Charvat, J.M., Limoli, C.L., et al, "Apollo Lunar Astronauts Show Higher Cardiovascular Disease Mortality: Possible Deep Space Radiation Effects on the Vascular Endothelium," *Scientific Reports 6*, July 28, 2016, 29901.

[128] Moll, Stephan,et al, "Venous Thrombosis during Spaceflight," *New England Journal of Medicine*, January 2, 2020; 382:89–90.

as are found in space. The irradiated animals developed inflammatory changes in the endothelial cells lining their blood vessels, confirming the connection. It would make for interesting research to repeat the mouse experiment, this time giving them B vitamers and/or anti-inflammatory medications before exposing them to radiation. I believe the anti-inflammatory actions of B_{12} and folate could possibly guard against some of the effects of radiation and reduce the endothelial cell inflammatory response, offering some protection to the circulatory system.

There is also the issue of weight. Despite the fact that menus are individualized for each astronaut and are rotated over six-to-ten days to provide variety, astronauts' appetites still drop over time. The decline could be due to weightlessness, motion sickness, radiation, the reality that food in space tastes bland, or some other unknown factor. In general, the longer the flight, the greater the appetite problem, and the greater the potential for subsequent nutritional deficiencies.

We have already seen space travelers having difficulty with weight and bone loss, vision, heart disease, and more. What else might go wrong? It's impossible to predict, but there's no reason to believe we have discovered all the potential health and nutrition problems, given we've only taken tiny steps away from our planet. If we are to expect astronauts to survive multiyear journeys into outer space, nutrition must become as important a subject as physics and astronomy. Future space travelers should have their genomes and biomes mapped to look for predispositions to illness and vitamer deficiencies. The proficiency of their vitamin-to-vitamer metabolism should be checked to see if they have adequate amounts of the MTHFR enzyme. If they do not, their emotional and physical health will suffer, and they won't be able to call in sick.

Just as a source of B_{12} from shellfish protected our species 100,000 years ago, the vitamers might again save us as we explore and settle beyond our planet. It is unlikely that explorers will perfect a way to store enough beef or oysters for long voyages or raise cows on Mars, so the main source of vitamers will be from supplementation. Every traveler should get enough B_{12}/folate tablets to last the length of the voyage.

Our current approach to nutrition for long-term space flight is to let the voyagers get most, if not all, of their nutrition from the food prepacked in the space pantry, with "special deliveries" arriving with the occasional supply ships. Each astronaut is also allowed to choose which supplements, if any, he or she wants to take while in space. The most recent exception to this rule is the requirement that vitamin D tablets be taken throughout the trip to prevent bone loss and other hormonal abnormalities. (Remember, all the vitamin D in the world will not prevent bone loss unless there is enough B12/F.) Does it make sense to rely on the individual astronaut's personal vitamin selection? Keep in mind, today's trips are not just for eight days, as the first moon landing was.

Hundreds of years ago, scurvy decimated sailing ships, killing thousands of sailors. Today's space program directors don't want their explorers to face a vitamin deficiency and disability any more than the British Admiralty wanted their eighteenth-century explorers to develop an easily preventable disease.

The Coming "Nutrition World War"

Space travel is exciting, filled with mystery and the hope of great discoveries. War is a different matter, a miserable one that is often linked to vitamers—specifically to their availability, or lack thereof.

Right about the time Rome ruled the Western world, there were around 400 million people walking the Earth. One thousand years later, that number, as a result of crowding, animal carried pathogens (plagues), and poor nutrition, had actually fallen to 345 million. By 1500 the world population had only climbed to 540 million. The number began rising dramatically as agricultural techniques improved and we moved into the Industrial Revolution, and by 1850 there were 1.2 billion men, women, and children on Earth. From this point, the numbers begin racing up the graph with frightening speed. We hit 3 billion in 1960, 4 billion in about 1975, and 5 billion in the late 1980s. Today's count is about 7 billion, and we're expected to hit 9 billion humans by the 2040s.

Unfortunately, we are not able to properly feed and nourish all the people we have now, for the land necessary to grow food and graze animals is limited, and the cost of land is going up while its availability is dropping. It takes a long time for new soil to be created—millions of years—but we've managed to use up almost all of it over the past one thousand years of intensive farming. Research conducted by the University of Sheffield's Grantham Centre for Sustainable Futures demonstrated that the land available to grow crops has decreased by 33 percent over the past two decades, thanks to intensive farming and ongoing climate change. The center notes that unless a worldwide program to preserve what we have left is developed and implemented, the results will be disastrous. One quick statistic says it all: According to a 2009 study published in the *Proceedings of the National Academy of Sciences of the*

United States of America, the yield of corn, soybeans, and cotton in the United States will decrease by 30 to 46 percent by the end of this century under the best of circumstances.[129]

Since we can't wait another 2 million or 10 million years for new soil to be created, we are dependent upon escalating amounts of fertilizers and pesticides to keep from falling further behind in our insatiable demand for food. Increasingly intensive forms of farming are terribly harmful to the land over the long run. Meanwhile, the energy and environmental costs of clearing fields, nourishing them, then harvesting and transporting animals and crops continues to rise.

Given the limits of our current food-growing and distribution techniques, plus the fact that many people still go to bed hungry each night, it seems as if the human population is approaching a critical sustainability level, beyond which we will not be able to feed many more. Thanks to the wealth and power disparities between nations, some countries are already suffering from widespread food shortages and mass migrations to places with more. The poorer populations—already forced to be involuntary vegans because they simply cannot afford meat—will have increased health challenges, further depleting resources. Unless various political groups get over their absolutism when it comes to international family planning, millions will be condemned at birth to die a horrible death from lack of water, food, and healthcare. Populations are now on the move just to survive.

Battle lines may have already been drawn; indeed, the opening salvo in this world struggle for nutrients was fired in the South China Sea. This large body of water, surrounded by China, Vietnam, the Philippines, and many other countries, is rich in fish to be shared by all, but disputed claims are being made for this resource. Among nations sharing their fishery statistics, it is known that fish populations in territorial waters are already seriously depleted. We have no comparable information regarding the fisheries of countries that choose to hide this information. The fact that fishing fleets are being sent farther and farther from their home waters strongly suggests that they are running out of local seafood nutrients, causing an increase in fish piracy.

People have to eat, there are more and more people to feed, and it is becoming more and more difficult—and costly—to feed everyone by growing plants or grazing animals. How many years will pass before unilateral

---

[129] Schlenker, W., Roberts, M.J., "Nonlinear Temperature Effects Indicate Severe Damages to U.S. Crop Yields Under Climate Change," *Proceedings of the National Academy of Sciences of the USA*, 2009; 106(37):15594–15598.

"land-grabs," "fish-grabs," and other aggressive moves lead to actual conflict?

Shifting Stresses

As if overpopulation, a looming shortage of soil, and potential wars over fishing rights weren't enough, we're also facing a reshuffling of some stressors as the environment evolves to our demands. Yes, changes in climate cause serious and difficult-to-predict changes in our stressors.

In recent years, for example, we've seen a non-biologic (abiotic) stress "turn into" biotic stress. A change in climate temperature is an abiotic stress in and of itself. That would be challenging enough to adapt to, but the environmental changes triggered by global warming are allowing certain viruses, bacteria, and parasites to move into new territories. This is already causing trouble as, for example, the Zika and Chikungunya viruses spread from South and Central America up into North America, where the temperature is becoming compatible with these dangerous pathogens.

Even as we become increasingly dependent on the ocean to provide for our nutritional needs, and as countries are edging closer to war over fishing rights, climate change is making eating fish a riskier proposition. Increased water temperatures triggered by climate transformation in some areas leads to longer breeding seasons for fish and shellfish-borne cholera bacteria. According to the Centers for Disease Control and Prevention, there has been almost a threefold increase in *Vibrio cholerae* infections from food and drinking water. This serious infection triggers severe intestinal symptoms and dehydration leading to death. Climate change has already been linked to an increased incidence of cholera in Alaska, of all places.[130]

In addition to dealing with the spread of existing viruses, bacteria, parasites, and the inevitable emergence of new ones, we will need to protect ourselves against natural toxins made by a variety of plants in response to their environmental stress. Diseases and toxins causing sickness in new geographic regions can certainly be considered "climate change illnesses," and abiotic stresses become biotic. This will require all the vitamers and modulators we can muster to fight them.

Meanwhile, climate changes are also hampering the ability of certain areas to grow abundant food as they did in the past. A 2016 study in the

---

[130] Veaaulli, L., Grande, C., Reid, P.C., et al, "Climate Influence on Vibrio and Associated Human Diseases During the Past Half-Century in the Coastal North Atlantic," *Proceedings of the National Academy of Sciences of the USA*, 2016; 113(34):E5062–E5071.

British medical journal The Lancet indicated that by 2050, global climate alteration will reduce nutritional health to such an extent that it will cause more than 500,000 deaths a year.[131] How many millions who aren't killed outright by faltering nutrition will instead suffer various physical and emotional ills?

The Backward-Creeping "Earth Overshoot Day"

Every year, the Global Footprint Network calculates the planet's biocapacity, which is our ability to produce renewable resources and food. This organization compares this biocapacity to our actual yearly consumption—are we are producing enough renewable resources to meet our needs each year? And if not, at what point in the year do we tip into a deficit?

If we produced exactly as much as we needed, that tipping point would be at the very end of the day on December 31. No deficit, no worries. If we only produced half as much as we needed, that date would be July 1—for the entire second half of the year, we'd be living (and eating) our way into trouble.

Unfortunately, we are doing just that. In 1987, "Earth Overshoot Day," or the day when yearly consumption outstripped yearly production, was December 19. That's not too far back; we made it almost to the end of the year. In 2009 Earth Overshoot Day was September 25, and in 2019 it was July 29th. It's as if the Earth is going into deficit earlier each year and living off its "credit cards" for longer periods of time. We are collectively out of homeostasis.

At this rate, sooner or later, credit will be shut off, and billions of people will suffer and die. Knowing this, shouldn't we more aggressively address the issue of resources versus consumption today, while there's still a reasonable chance of preventing such misery?

Another major "shifting stress," as mentioned in earlier chapters, is air pollution. We've long understood that this is a serious problem, contributing

---

[131] Springmann, M., et al, "Global and Regional Health Effects of Future Food Production Under Climate Change: A Modelling Study," *The Lancet*, 2016; 387(10031):1937–1946.

to lung disease, heart disease, and more. In a talk titled "The Global Burden of Disease from Air Pollution" presented to the American Association for the Advancement of Science in 2016, Michael Brauer stated that in 2013, air pollution led to 5.5 million premature deaths worldwide.[132] Air pollution was the fourth leading cause of death, with most of these deaths occurring in India and China. Dr. Bauer pointed out that death by air pollution is manifested in increased rates of heart disease, stroke, lung cancer, bronchitis, emphysema, and infections, all of which are inflammation-related illnesses. This occurrence, found all over the world, can be seen as a form of unintended, painful population control.

Air pollution is a stressor in and of itself, but now, as new forms of pollution are entering the environment, they are triggering new stresses. For example, by-product nanoparticles have joined other air pollutants in recent years, and they are being found in the brain tissue of people suffering with Alzheimer's disease.[133] If we extrapolate our new knowledge of inflammation response, it makes sense these particles could be causing micro-inflammatory sites the brain responds to by putting down the neuro-plaques found in Alzheimer's patients. As in the agouti mice exposed to BPA, vitamers might offer some protection.

If Not Meatless, Then Less Meat

Many modern humans have a complex relationship with meat, believing it is detrimental for them, or somehow objectionable, yet feeling a powerful urge to eat it. Humans are programmed to eat meat; we have a drive to replenish our stores of vitamin B12 and folate. If you doubt it, consider that when people are deprived of nutrients for financial, medical, or surgical reasons, they may develop a disorder called pica. People with this condition are driven to search out nutrients by eating soil, clay, stones, glass, and other substances as their bodies attempt to capture them. A similar nutrient drive can be seen in vegans who describe having dysphoric meat-craving dreams—"meatmares."

---

[132] Brauer, Michael, "The Global Burden of Disease from Air Pollution," *AAAS 2016 Annual Meeting*, February 13, 2016.

[133] Heusinkveld, H.J., Wahle, T., Campbell, A., et al, "Neurodegenerative and Neurological Disorders by Small Inhaled Particles, *NeuroToxicology*, 2016; 56:94–106.

Dreaming of Beef?

One of my patients became Hindu and developed strong convictions against eating red meat. Several months after his conversion, I asked him if he had any "red meat" dreams. His answer was enlightening: He said he had never had one, because even dreaming of eating red meat would be objectionable. After some thought, he said he was having dreams about eating chicken livers. This nutrient-rich food was, unconsciously, more acceptable to him than red-meat dreams, and his sleeping mind intuitively knew what food was high in B12 and folate. When I started him on B vitamer supplements, the "chicken-liver" dreams went away.

I believe that when the body has an abundant supply of B12 and folate vitamers via supplementation, the primitive evolutionary urges pushing us to seek out red meat can be significantly reduced. I've had many patients describe a natural and easy reduction in their craving for and consumption of beef when they started taking vitamers. This vitamer-driven reduction in the desire for meat protein would certainly be a boon for those embarking on a years-long mission to Mars. It would also be appealing to those who wish to reduce their meat consumption for ethical, religious, or environmental concerns.

Man-Made Meat

The most expensive foods in the grocery store or on a restaurant menu are usually the umami-rich proteins, our best sources of B12 and folate. We probably developed that additional umami taste sense to seek out such sources. Meat of all kinds will only become increasingly expensive as time passes, which means that future generations all over the world could end up being voluntary or involuntary vegans.

Artificial meat and fish proteins have long been on the horizon, and it is now being created so we might have an option for a reduced meat-dependent future. It makes no sense to make a "burger" to replace beef when the thing we are biologically attracted to in a burger through umami is the vitamers. It is absolutely necessary that B12 and folate be part of the artificial meat/fish recipe. Otherwise, meatless protein will not reduce the natural human drive to consume meat and will not confer its benefits.

If the use of vitamers becomes widespread and results in a global reduction in the urge to consume meat and fish, even by 10 percent, we could significantly reduce the strain on the planet and begin to push back the clock on Earth Overshoot Day. Less land would be devoted to the production of red meat, meaning less pollution, less use of livestock antibiotics, less energy expended to convert cattle into hamburgers, and more land available for other practices. Lightening the environmental load on the planet, as well as the inflammatory load on all of us, would be a boon for both our planetary and individual health.

B-Fortified

Few of us are astronauts, and here in the United States most of us still eat red meat when we choose, yet some still suffer from a vitamer deficiency. It may be time to fortify certain foods with vitamer B12 as has been done in some countries with folate. B12 and folate-fortification has been recommended by nutrition experts who now realize that B12 deficiency is more prominent and causes more disability than does folate deficiency.

Jane E. Brody, the noted *New York Times* health columnist and dean of health and wellness journalism, has been writing about B12 deficiency for many years. She eloquently described the concerns about the lack of B12 in her article titled "A Push for Adding B12, Though the Jury is Still Out," which was written way back in 2008. In her article she quoted Dr. Godfrey Oakley, a proponent of fortification, as saying, "If B12 were required in flour, the problem of low stomach acid would essentially disappear," and it would reduce the risk of people "developing dementia, osteoporosis and cardiovascular disease."[134] In Brody's more recent B12 article, "Vitamin B12 as Protection for the Aging Brain," dated September 6, 2016, she notes the importance of adequate B12 and folate for slowing cognitive decline. (*Jane Brody's Nutrition Book*, written in 1988, still holds up well.)

---

[134] Oakley, G.P., Tulchinsky, T. H., "Folic Acid and Vitamin B12 Fortification of Flour: A Global Basic Food Security Requirement," *Public Health Reviews*, 2010; 32(1):284–295.

Shelf Life-Less

How fortified grain products are stored can make all the difference in whether there are sufficient synthetic vitamins available for absorption and conversion. When fortified flour is shipped and stored in standard paper bags for longer than six months, 50 percent or more of the folic acid, and cyanocobalamin when added, decompose to the point of significantly reduced nutritional value.[135]

Better, Less-Expensive Health

We've tackled an important topic in this book—the confluence of decreasing vitamers, poor epigenetic methylation, and the resultant effects of an increasing inflammatory load on the body. I hope I've convinced laypeople and physicians to take another look at the need for B vitamins and to be concerned about the specific vitamer form in which these essential nutrients are sold to the public.

I believe that simply ensuring that everyone gets enough of these vitamers would radically alter some aspects of medical practice for the better, producing more cost-effective treatments for many ailments and better health for us all. I hope a reevaluation of many different medical procedures and treatment protocols will soon take place, with the standard of care being expanded to include B12/F vitamer supplementation. This could apply to a variety of medical situations, including:

- Diabetics at risk for peripheral neuropathy and heart disease
- Post-gastric bypass surgery
- Patients taking birth control pills and hormone replacement therapy
- Patients taking gastric acid reduction (GERD) medications
- Patients receiving repeated doses of nitrous oxide
- Diabetics taking blood-sugar reduction medication
- Vegans and vegetarians (voluntary and involuntary)
- Patients overindulging in alcohol use

---

[135] Hemery, Y., et al, "Influence of Storage Conditions and Packaging of Fortified Wheat Flour on Microbial Load and Stability of Folate and Vitamin B12, Food Chemistry: X, December 14, 2019.

- Patients being treated for AIDS/HIV
- Patients with a MTHFR deficiency
- Obstetric patients at risk for maternal thromboembolism, post-partum depression
- Patients with a BMI in the unhealthy range
- Patients with cognitive decline
- Patients with burn injuries
- Children at risk for autism and developmental delays
- Patients undergoing major surgery, orthopedic surgery, or reconstructive surgery
- Infertility treatment (both women and men)
- Patients receiving psychiatric medications
- Patients at risk for cancer of the cervix, prostate, colon, or breast
- All earthlings going to Mars

Vitamer Therapeutics Education

I also hope that in the near future, medical appointments will include proactive nutrition counseling covered by insurance companies. In some medical school programs, the educators are ahead of the curve and have included formal culinary medicine programs based upon the model set up at Tulane University Medical School. There they have made learning about how nutrients get into the body and how they are utilized just as important as studying anatomy and biochemistry.

The widespread lack of concern about nutrient nutrition is a shared responsibility. Overworked physicians and their staff are inundated just trying to take care of the immediate complaints bringing people to their office. Patients too often ignore any nutritional advice they get from their physicians. We need all parties—insurance companies, physicians, and patients—to embrace the health-building properties of the vitamers and other nutrients.

You now have the knowledge to interpret news reports from the field of medicine as studies are posted. When a report states there is an increased risk for stomach cancer in those taking PPIs for GERD symptoms, you'll know that a contributing mechanism is B12/F deficiency. When you see research about the increased risk of blood clots in post-menopausal women taking estrogen and progesterone, you'll know about the process of B12/F deficiency. When you hear about children at increased risk for developmental delays and autism in countries that don't have B vitamin-fortification, you will know the reason before anyone else. When a news report states that vegan women are more at risk for pulmonary embolism, you will know the B12/F deficiency connection.[136] When you hear that women with higher BMIs have an increased risk of cancer, heal poorly from burns, and respond inadequately to vaccines, you'll have the knowledge that low folate is the common cause.

A Closing Word or Two

As you have learned by reading this book, vitamers are vital to our health and the health of the planet. I have endeavored to take three complex subjects—epigenetics, inflammation, and vitamer biochemistry—and present a case for understanding their critical interdependence. We have seen how vitamers were essential for our evolutionary progress and are essential for our advancement into the future.

Whether or not we think about the topics of overpopulation, pollution, and climate change, we are all dealing with the consequences. The onslaught of manipulated foods turns our bodies into excess adipose tissue depositories. Facing these challenges head-on with the help of vitamers as one of many modulators will make for a healthier outcome for more people, allowing the reallocation of resources toward the other life-threatening trials to come. Adenosyl-B12, methyl-B12, and folate are no longer curiosities just for those who study nutrition—they are vital components of the healthy lives and longevity deserved by all.

---

[136] Chatzivasiloglou, F., et al, "Vegan Diet as an Indirect Risk Factor for Pulmonary Embolism," *Nutrients*, March 2019; 11(3):557.

BIBLIOGRAPHY

The following is a list of books I used as references and suggest for those who want a more in-depth view of the interconnection of epigenetics, inflammation, and vitamers:

Allen, John S. *The Omnivorous Mind: Our Evolving Relationship with Food.* Boston: Harvard University Press, 2012.

Braly, James, and Holford, Patrick. *The H-Factor Solution: Homocysteine, the Best Single Indicator of Whether You Are Likely to Live Long or Die Young.* North Bergren, NJ: Basic Health Publications, 2003.

Brody, Jane. *Jane Brody's Nutrition Book.* New York: Bantam, 1988.

Bronowski, Jacob. *The Ascent of Man.* London: The Folio Society, 2012.

Carey, Nessa. *The Epigenetics Revolution: How Modern Biology Is Rewriting Our Understanding of Genetics, Disease, and Inheritance.* New York: Columbia University Press, 2013.

Cass, Hyla. *Supplement Your Prescription: What Your Doctor Doesn't Know about Nutrition.* Portland, Or.: Basic Health Publications, 2009.

Combs, Gerald F., and McClung, James P. *The Vitamins: Fundamental Aspects in Nutrition and Health.* London: Elsevier, 2017.

Cooney, Craig, and Lawren, Bill. *Methyl Magic: Maximum Health through Methylation.* Kansas City: Andrews McNeel Pub, 1999.

Daruna, J. H. *Introduction to Psychoneuroimmunology*. Amsterdam: Elsevier, 2012.

Haslberger, Alexander G., and Gressler, Sabine, editors. *Epigenetics and Human Health: Linking Hereditary, Environmental and Nutritional Aspects.* Weinheim, Germany:Wiley-VCH, 2010.

Hendler, Sheldon Saul, and Rorvik, David M. *PDR for Nutritional Supplements.* Montvale, NJ: Thomson Reuters, 2008.

Lee, Sang-Hee, and Yoon, Shin-Young. *Close Encounters with Humankind: A Paleoanthropologist Investigates Our Evolving Species.* New York: W.W. Norton, 2019.

Ludwig, David. *Always Hungry? Conquer Cravings, Retrain Your Fat Cells, and Lose Weight Permanently.* New York: Grand Central Life & Style, 2018.

McCully, Kilmer S. *The Homocysteine Revolution: Medicine for the New Millennium.* Los Angeles: Keats Pub, 1999.

Meller, William. *Evolution Rx: A Practical Guide to Harnessing Our Innate Capacity for Health and Healing.* New York: Penguin Group, 2010.

Pacholok, Sally M., and Stuart, Jeffrey J. *Could It Be B12? An Epidemic of Misdiagnoses.* Chicago: Linden Publishing, 2011.

Panda, Satchin. *The Circadian Code: Lose Weight, Supercharge Your Energy, and Transform Your Health from Morning to Midnight.* New York: Rodale, an imprint of the Crown Publishing Group, 2018.

Faith, Robert E., Murgo, Anthony, J., et al. *Cytokines: Stress and Immunity.* Boca Raton: Taylor & Francis Group, 2007.

Pollan, Michael. *Food Rules: An Eater's Manual.* New York: Penguin Books, 2013.

Price, Catherine. *Vitamania: Our Obsessive Quest for Nutritional Perfection.* New York: Penguin Press, 2015.

Rio, Linda M. *The Hormone Factor in Mental Health: Bridging the Mind-Body Gap*. London: Jessica Kingsley, 2014.

Siegel, Allan, and Zalcman, Steven S. *The Neuroimmunological Basis of Behavior and Mental Disorders*. New York: Springer Science Business Media, 2009.

Talbott, Shawn. *Cortisol Connection: Why Stress Makes You Fat and Ruins Your Health—and What You Can Do About It*. Alameda, Calif.: Hunter House, Inc., 2007.

Tattersall, Ian. *Masters of the Planet: Seeking the Origins of Human Singularity*. New York: Palgrave Macmillan, 2012.

Wrangham, Richard. *Catching Fire: How Cooking Made Us Human*. New York: Basic Books, 2010.

Lee, Sang-Hee, and Yoon, Shin-Young. *Close Encounters with Humankind: A Paleoanthropologist Investigates Our Evolving Species*. New York: W.W. Norton, 2019.

Zinczenko, David, & Moore, Peter. (2015). *The 8 Hour Diet: Watch the Pounds Disappear Without Watching What You Eat!* New York: Rodale, 2013.

AFTERWORD

The science of vitamers, epigenetics, and inflammation is always progressing. If you have an interest in the ongoing developments in the field of vitamer dynamics, log on to sheldonzablowmd.com. On the website, I will review current research and news articles that note the medical benefits of B vitamers. The site will also note if and when good vitamer supplements become available.

ACKNOWLEDGMENTS

This complex project would not have been possible without the help of many, but primary among them is my editor Barry Fox. He patiently guided this first-time book author from the beginning in 2013 when I only had two graphs to show him. I sweated every draft he said I could do better. The support, patience, and grammatical eye of my wife, Lorna, were almost infinite, as were the times I said, "I just finished the final draft."

Anthony Wagner has been a steadfast friend through the ups and downs of this journey, and his support has been essential. I owe many thanks to Gary Friedman, who was one of the first people to listen and encourage me to proceed with the science behind the book.

There were two close friends who read the earliest draft, Dan Pearson (*Marañón* Chocolates) and Tammy Sirotenko, who offered their encouragement when I needed it the most. I would like to thank two science editors, Tiffany Fox and Janet Lockett, for their contributions, as well as Colette Freedman for her valued suggestions. My thanks also go to Steve Cook, who patiently put my ideas into the graphics that are used in the book. A shout-out also goes to Libby Kingsbury, who also aided in the production of charts for use. Thanks go to Jonathan Pleska for his work on the cover art.

On the literary side, my first thanks goes to Greg Reid (author/film producer), who was kind in encouraging me and putting me in contact with Gary Krebs (author/agent). Gary then had me connect with Karen Strauss at Hybrid Global Publishing, who took the project from there. Her guidance and support was crucial in pulling everything together. With the aid and patience of her assistants, Claudia Volkman and Sara Foley, the book was finalized. A special thanks to my close friend Allen Karp for his suggestions, sharp eye, and helping me with my writer's proofreading blindness.

Finally, I would like to thank my patients, who have taught me so much through their courage and resilience and schooled me on how to explain complex matters in less complex ways.

INDEX

Note: (ill.) indicates photos and illustrations.

CPSIA information can be obtained
at www.ICGtesting.com
Printed in the USA
LVHW082345161020
668889LV00010B/236